Wounded

Wounded

A New History of the Western Front in World War I

EMILY MAYHEW

OXFORD
UNIVERSITY PRESS

OXFORD

UNIVERSITY PRESS

Oxford University Press is a department of the University of Oxford.
It furthers the University's objective of excellence in research,
scholarship, and education by publishing worldwide.

Oxford   New York

Auckland   Cape Town   Dar es Salaam   Hong Kong   Karachi
Kuala Lumpur   Madrid   Melbourne   Mexico City   Nairobi
New Delhi   Shanghai   Taipei   Toronto

With offices in

Argentina   Austria   Brazil   Chile   Czech Republic   France   Greece
Guatemala   Hungary   Italy   Japan   Poland   Portugal   Singapore
South Korea   Switzerland   Thailand   Turkey   Ukraine   Vietnam

Oxford is a registered trade mark of Oxford University Press
in the UK and certain other countries.

Published in the United States of America by
Oxford University Press
198 Madison Avenue, New York, NY 10016

First issued as an Oxford University Press paperback, 2016

First published in Great Britain in 2013 by
The Bodley Head

Library of Congress Cataloging-in-Publication Data
Mayhew, E. R. (Emily R.)
Wounded : a new history of the Western Front in World War I / Emily Mayhew.
pages   cm
Includes bibliographical references and index.
ISBN 978-0-19-932245-9 (hardcover); 978-0-19-045444-9 (paperback)
1. World War, 1914–1918—Medical care—Great Britain—Case studies.
2. World War, 1914–1918—Medical care—Europe, Western—Case studies.
3. Great Britain. Army—Medical care—History—20th century.
4. Medicine, Military—Great Britain—History—20th century. I. Title.
D629.G7M19   2013
940.4'7541—dc23   2013016329

Contents

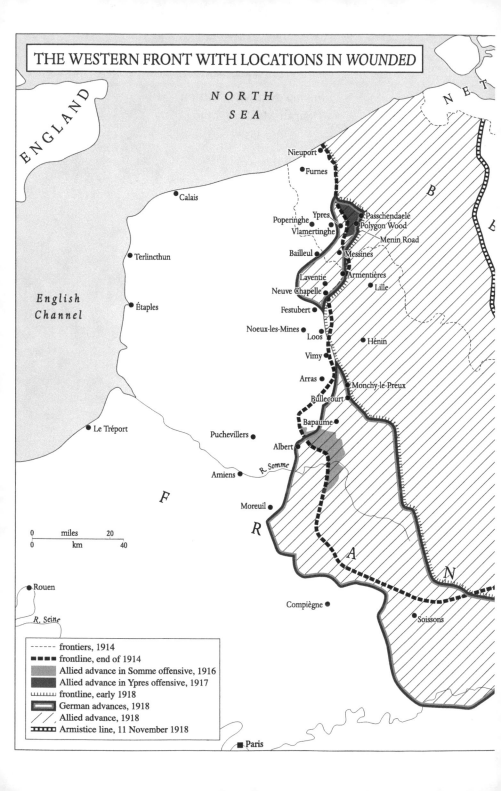

THE WESTERN FRONT WITH LOCATIONS IN *WOUNDED*

ENGLAND

NORTH SEA

NET

B

B

Calais

Nieuport
• Furnes

Ypres • • Passchendaele
Poperinghe • Polygon Wood
Vlamertinghe
Menin Road
Bailleul • • Messines
Laventie • Armentières
Neuve Chapelle • Lille
Festubert •
Noeux-les-Mines • Loos
• Hénin
Vimy •
Arras • • Monchy-le-Preux
Bullecourt •
Bapaume •
Albert •
Amiens •   R. Somme
Moreuil •

Terlincthun •

English
Channel

Étaples •

Le Tréport •

Puchevillers •

F

R

A

N

• Rouen

R. Seine

Compiègne •

• Soissons

0	miles	20
0	km	40

----- frontiers, 1914
▄▄▄▄ frontline, end of 1914
▒▒▒ Allied advance in Somme offensive, 1916
▓▓▓ Allied advance in Ypres offensive, 1917
ɯɯɯ frontline, early 1918
▭ German advances, 1918
/// Allied advance, 1918
▰▰▰ Armistice line, 11 November 1918

■ Paris

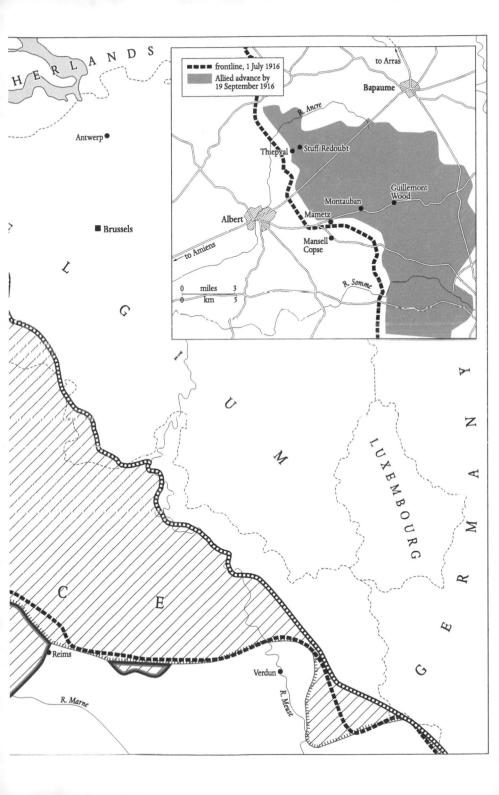

HERLANDS

Antwerp ●

■ Brussels

L

G

frontline, 1 July 1916

Allied advance by
19 September 1916

to Arras

Bapaume

R. Ancre

Thiepval ● ● Stuff Redoubt

Albert

to Amiens

● Montauban

Guillemont
Wood

Mametz

Mansell
Copse

0   miles   3
0   km   5

R. Somme

I

U

M

LUXEMBOURG

G

E

R

M

A

N

Y

C

E

Reims ●

Verdun ●

R. Marne

R. Meuse

Introduction

Being wounded was one of the most common experiences of the Great War. On the Western Front, almost every other British soldier could expect to become a casualty, with physical injuries ranging in severity from light wounds to permanent, life-changing disabilities. Yet in the historical record of the First World War, the wounded and the men and women who cared for them are an undiscovered, somehow silenced group. As readers of Great War history, we have become accustomed to the noise of the blasting, thumping barrage and the shrieks of officers' whistles ordering the men over the top. We are much less accustomed to the sounds of the voices of the wounded. The scale and power of the fighting has drowned them out. But their stories deserve to be heard and understood – just as we have learned to listen to the words of the war poets – for everything they can tell us about suffering and war.

Much of what we do know about the wounded of the First World War comes from writers of fiction. Bestselling books such as *Birdsong* and *Regeneration* tell beautiful and moving stories of casualties, nurses and doctors, and the extraordinary play *War Horse* is set at a medical aid post where Joey and Topthorn pull ambulances. These works are based on detailed historical research but they are not – nor are they intended to be – history. *Wounded* is about the real men and women who inspired these writers. It is a work of historical rediscovery but it is not a conventional history. Like a novel, it uses a continuous narrative to interweave the testimonies of injured soldiers and stretcher bearers, doctors and surgeons, nurses and chaplains, orderlies and hospital train staff, and volunteers in train stations in France and Britain. By bringing together all these different voices for the first time, the book guides the reader through the world of the wounded and those who cared for them.

Writing *Wounded* in this unconventional way was not simply a question of preference for one representational style over another. As I researched the book, I came to realise that the only choice I had as a historian was to tell the story unconventionally – or not tell it at all. The conventional approach would require an analysis of the official archive of military medical operations during the Great War to create a comprehensive overview of the planning and process of medical care. Policy documents from the War Office would be meshed with implementation reports from the Army Medical Services. Treasury financial records would coordinate with Royal Army Medical Corps staffing reports. Hospital archives would align with casualty statistics. Finally, some personal testimony would be added to provide colour and human detail to the history of the huge operational undertaking. Yet such a conventional approach proved impossible, for one simple reason: very few of those documents are still available. Most of the material that was in the national archives relating to the medical conduct of the war is gone; what is left is at best partial. In the mid-1920s no one could think of a reason to keep the mass of official documents relating to such a relatively narrow aspect of the war, so no one did.

Thus the history had to be written with what was left, and it turned out that what was left was enough. I began to gather testimonies of individuals, most of them unpublished, and bring them together in a collective narrative. Some were tucked into a file in an archive, faded and almost forgotten; some were just a page or a fragment from a hastily scribbled letter home. Others were well-organised, neatly written accounts spanning the entire course of the war. There was the rough and unschooled voice of the stretcher bearer and the smooth, educated prose of the surgeon's memoir. Nurses' diaries told of the dreadful nights when they were almost overwhelmed by casualties coming to them straight from the Somme, but also of how they coped living so close to the war. Orderlies wrote of the unexpected moments of happiness they experienced – moments that could confound them as much as the never-ending violence of the front. Some of the most valuable testimony came from a group without previous medical training or experience: the army chaplains who took on new and unexpected roles in hospitals, aid posts, and sometimes on the battlefield, as they tried to find ways of offering service in a place of suffering. Bringing all these voices together I began to assemble a history of the central experience that was repeated hundreds of thousands of times up and down the Western Front and went beyond rank or status: the wounding of a soldier and the struggle of medics to save his life.

And then there are the voices of the wounded themselves. Each of the chapters in this book tells an individual story (and sometimes a number of stories) but collectively they follow the path taken by the wounded soldier: his journey from injury on the battlefield to recovery in a hospital in Britain. The wounded spent a surprising amount of time on the move during their medical treatment, and to many their first journey felt like the longest of all. To survive they had to get off and away from the battlefield. Sometimes they travelled on a stretcher, sometimes on the back of a comrade and sometimes they were on their own, crawling a few feet at a time to find help at the aid post. There the Regimental Medical Officer tried to make sure they could survive the next leg of the journey – from aid post to casualty clearing station. Here they met the nurses who would resuscitate them and the surgeons who would operate on their wounds. For some, this was the end of their journey. Either they went back to their battalion or they took the shorter path to the moribund ward and then to the cemetery, where they would be buried by the chaplain.

For those too ill to return to duty, there was another journey to take and another world to discover. The medical system relied on trains to move large numbers of wounded around France and back home to Britain. These journeys could last for days. Hospital trains had the lowest priority on the rails, after troop, ammunition and supply trains. They waited in sidings for hours, sometimes days, for other trains to pass by, and then slowly made their way north to the coast. They were called 'hospital trains' for a reason: each carriage was a ward full of patients, cared for by nurses and orderlies for however long the journey took.

Travel by hospital train had a flaw. Long delays meant connections missed and the wounded soldier detrained at stations in both France and Britain often found that no one was waiting for him. His journey stopped in a dark, chilly terminus, where he might lie throughout the night unattended on a concrete platform until the system got working again and he was moved on. Medical officials were never able to get to grips with this disconnection but all over France, and in London, individuals did their best to solve the problem independently. If he was lucky, the wounded soldier would meet one of these volunteers on a platform while he waited. It might be a nurse taking mugs of hot soup and sandwiches round on trays, or one of the indefatigable volunteers of the London Ambulance Column at a mainline London station who made sure the wounded soldier got to his destination – a hospital bed in Blighty – quickly and with as little pain as possible.

The focus of *Wounded* is the British Army on the Western Front. Here the military medical system faced its greatest challenge, failed and was rebuilt. In 1914 the Army's medical staff had been installed in a well-organised network of base hospitals, newly fitted out in towns and cities well away from the front. They were experienced; many had served in South Africa and in Britain's other colonial wars and felt they knew what to expect. But then the first soldier arrived on their operating table and they realised that everything they knew about treating casualties was useless.

So in early 1915, after the offensives slowed, with both sides gasping for breath and facing each other in hundreds of miles of trenches, the medical services began to adjust to the new war and its new wounds.

The Flanders casualty was almost torn apart. Gone were the neat round holes made by rounded ammunition that flew slowly in the hot, dry African sun, could be easily located and extracted, and didn't leave much damage behind. Instead, the cylindro-conical bullet fired by the new powerful weaponry hit fast and hard, went deep and took bits of dirty uniform and airborne soil particles with it. Inside the human body, it ricocheted off bones and ploughed through soft tissue until its energy was spent. Shrapnel fragments were just as bad. They created jagged wounds, huge blooms of trauma that didn't stop bleeding and, if the casualty could survive long enough, provided the perfect environment for infection and sepsis. And there were so many of them. At the base hospitals soldier after soldier arrived with the most dreadful injuries: deep, ragged wounds to their heads, faces, limbs and abdomens.

In France the medics realised that there was no point having a well-organised network of hospitals with bright modern operating theatres full of lights and antiseptic procedures if none of their patients survived long enough to get there. Too many men bled to death or died of shock before their ambulance was even halfway to the hospital. Speed was vital. The journey from wounding to treatment had to be made as short and as quick as possible. There was only one way to do that: surgeons and hospitals would have to get closer to the wounded.

In the first months of 1915, with the Western Front fixed in the position it would hold until the last few months of the war, the entire British military medical system moved. Leaving their well-equipped base hospitals behind, surgeons set up units as close to the battlefield as they could get. They weren't starting entirely from scratch. There were medical facilities already there – the casualty clearing stations. They were tented and equipped to provide dressing changes and drinks to casualties, but they were run by teams of qualified medical officers and nurses and were easily adapted. And although no one thought to change their name, within months these casualty clearing stations became fully staffed, fully equipped hospitals in the field where the wounded could get to them quickly and directly. It turned out that it didn't matter that the surgeons were operating in a wooden hut or a canvas tent in earshot of the guns, or that improvisation was often the order of the day. What mattered was that they and their staff were close and undaunted so that lives were saved that would otherwise have been lost.

But it wasn't quite enough. Although hospitals had been brought close to the battlefield, casualties were still dying before they could reach them. Advanced first aid for the serious casualties needed to happen sooner – as close to the moment and place of wounding as possible. As with the casualty clearing stations, the solution was already there but it needed significant adaptation. At the beginning of the war, stretcher bearers were seen as little more than donkeys. All the qualification they needed was to be strong enough to pick up the wounded and move them to wherever they could be given treatment. This had to change. A dedicated stretcher-bearer corps was created. Bearers were specially recruited and trained in advanced first aid, including the vital skill of controlling haemorrhages. They became the very first step in the care for the wounded, finding and treating them where they fell in the middle of the fighting. In under a year, and in time for the battle of the Somme, a new and essential medical trade was created on the Western Front.

Although a century has passed, and wars have been transformed, the British system for caring for its wounded remains the same: its primary component is the clinically capable forward surgical facility. Today's field hospitals are more accurately named than casualty clearing stations, but they are based on the models conceived by the medics of the Western Front. The field hospital at Camp Bastion in Afghanistan looks and operates very much like its predecessors in the Great War. It is located as close to the fighting as possible. It can be adapted instantly to meet the needs of the incoming casualties. It is staffed by extraordinary men and women who drive it forward by their courage and ingenuity. And the stretcher-bearer corps has its direct descendants, too. The men and women of the Medical Emergency Response Teams (MERT) know how to find and treat a wounded soldier whilst under attack. While they may arrive by helicopter, they also use their special skills and training to save lives and keep them saved, no matter what the journey.

Author's Note

For readers wanting to engage more closely with the world of the wounded, the notes and references at the back of the book list the primary sources I have used and provide an overview of the academic context for medical care during the Great War. Readers will also find a timeline which puts the story of *Wounded* into the context of the general history of the war. The notes for each chapter also include a short list of relevant poems and paintings from the period that relate directly to the material presented in the text. All the works can be found in standard anthologies or online.

A note on the subtitle. 'Blighty' is a word of Hindu origin, being the anglicized form of the Indian word *vilayti*, meaning European or foreign. It became commonly used by British troops in India to refer to something from England, that is, from home. When regiments from India were sent to France, they brought the word with them and it entered general army slang. It acquired a particular meaning on the Western Front where a 'Blighty wound' or 'Blighty one' meant that an injury was so severe that the sufferer was certain to be sent home either for treatment or medical discharge. The word is still used in the British Army today.

I

Wounded

Mickey Chater, Neuve Chapelle, 12 March 1915

> I'm not one of those adventurous sportsmen who are always up for
> this kind of thing but I am convinced that it is the plain duty of
> every man who can, to go out if one is called upon . . . I am sure
> it would be a most splendid experience for those who come back.
>
> Mickey Chater, 3 August 1914

Somewhere along the Boulogne road the motor ambulance
bumped and jolted awake the young soldier hanging on a stretcher
in the rear. Other ruts and more bumping kept him conscious
and he tried to remember who he was and what had happened
to him. Then more lurching, and all that mattered was the terrible
pain that burned out from his face and took over his body and
mind. A steady piece of road gave him some breathing space,
enough to gather himself and focus on something else. When he
tried to open his eyes to see where he was, only one eye would
open; the other was stuck shut with something. As he tried to lift
his head, the pain tore through him again, so he lay back and
tried to breathe calmly, looking up at the ambulance roof of
narrow wooden slats and peeling paint spattered with blood, some
dried and old, some redder and fresh. It couldn't all have come
from him. Then another rut threw the ambulance into the air,
the soldier almost bumping his nose against the bloody roof.
Instinct made him turn his head away, but the movement brought
back the pain, and darkness engulfed him again. Just before he

lost consciousness he heard other cries in the ambulance. He realised he was not alone.

With the soldier silent, the ambulance struggled on. The driver would have been grateful for the moments of quiet, with none of the howling that had accompanied him from the minute he started the engine and pulled away from the ruined farmhouse that served as a medical post. He had tried to keep the ambulance steady, avoiding the holes and ruts in a road that had been chewed up by hundreds of other vehicles, horses and gun carriages going towards the battle of Neuve Chapelle, as well as scores of other ambulances going back and forth between the front and the hospitals at the coast.[1]

The driver realised that whatever he did made the howling worse. If he went faster, he hit the ruts harder and the ambulance bumped a foot or more into the air, before crashing down on its thin rubber tyres. But if he went slower, the vehicle might get stuck and would have to be pushed out. And slowing down only emphasised all the smaller bumps in the road. He had watched the men being loaded – broken and soaked in mud and gore – and, like all the other ambulance drivers, he knew he needed to drive fast. The hospitals were too far away from the battlefield and he didn't think the wounded men had enough blood in them to survive. So he accelerated away again. As the cries rose up from the back, he pressed his face close to the dirty windscreen and tried harder to find a piece of road with no craters, praying that they would be there soon.[2]

When the soldier regained consciousness he remembered who and where he was. He had fought at Neuve Chapelle, with the Gordons, and his name was Mickey Chater. He had been woken early on the first day of the battle by men creeping into the forward trenches; then there had been the sound of clanking metal and a faint smell of stew as their hot meal was passed around, amid hushed, nervy chatter. However much he had hoped to be joining them, he would not be. Instead he went to his battalion post to the rear to resume the work of digging relief trenches that his men had been doing all week.[3] Then, at first light, they heard clattering as gun crews wheeled pieces of artillery past them to get into position for the barrage that signalled the beginning of the battle.

At 07.30 the guns crashed into life and it seemed to Chater that the noise rang in his ears even now, as he lay in the ambulance. He had never heard anything like it. They had to stop work as both air and earth became one quivering jelly.[4] He remembered squadrons of aircraft flying overhead, and larks – hundreds of them, screaming a kind of frantic song as they were scared off the fields surrounding the town of Neuve Chapelle. He was surprised that even now he could still hear them above the thundering in his memory. Then the Gordons had watched the town being destroyed. Chater remembered seeing the trees that had lined the town square being blasted into the air, with broken boughs and branches landing pell-mell amongst the rubble. Shells hit a brewery, blowing it apart and sending hundreds of empty wooden barrels thumping down the streets. Soon he couldn't see the town any more through the clouds of dust. Everyone agreed that nothing could have survived the shelling. At 08.00 the soldiers went in.

Within an hour or so reports reached the Gordons that the forward troops' advance had been quick and successful; progress would continue to be made for three hours that morning. But then the reports began to change. First, returning artillery officers told of finding the town's cemetery blasted open, spilling corpses that had been buried there after the British Expeditionary Force's (BEF's) first desperate defence of the area six months earlier. It had to be a bad omen. Then the British advance slowed and stopped altogether in late morning. There was so much rubble in the town that troops were finding it difficult to make their way forward. They found themselves shelled by their own artillery, and all contact with the reserves who waited somewhere on the flanks had been lost.[5] Telephone cables were cut in more than fifty places.[6] And then the walking wounded began to emerge from the dust clouds. Chater and the Gordons broke off from their digging to help them sit down and to find them water. They learned that most of the enemy's barbed wire had survived the barrage, as had their snipers and camouflaged machine-gun nests, and the Germans were cutting men down like wheat at harvest time.

In the afternoon the Gordons saw a force of Royal Engineers advance towards the town to help fortify the place. Apart from the steady stream of stretchered wounded, no significant numbers of troops came back, so the Gordons assumed that those who had taken the town were holding on. By late afternoon it had become too dark to fight and things went quiet. Chater and his battalion thought they would be rested until morning, but an officer dashed over and ordered them out onto the battlefield to dig a new communications trench. The work took all night and was as back-breaking as it was demoralising, for all around them burial parties were retrieving uncountable numbers of corpses. It was dawn when they clambered back into their trenches for a quick meal and to await orders. As the sun came up, it showed the town wreathed in mist. There was no sign of the enemy.

The Gordons were ordered to join a regiment of Grenadier Guards and lined up for the attack. There were rumours that so many shells had been used the day before that, for the second morning of the battle, each gun had been allocated only five rounds. It was indeed a much shorter artillery barrage, and Chater barely had time to nod acknowledgements to those around him – some friends, some strangers – in the forward trench. Then shouted orders and whistles signalled the advance, the trench ladders went up and the men went over. In his ambulance, Chater tried to remember what had happened after that, but it would not come to him. His memory, sharp and clear until the very point of seeing his own muddied hands gripping the sides of the wooden trench ladder, failed him.

Perhaps it failed because, for the remainder of his battle of Neuve Chapelle, Chater would have been operating on raw instinct, trying to survive, with no time for thinking, and with the terrifying sound of the enemy artillery barrage coming closer and closer. Later he would remember that he pressed on, one boot in front of the other, trying to find a foothold in the rubble of stone, metal and splintered wood. And it was freezing – his hands white and numb gripping his rifle, and his breath puffing out like dragon smoke. Then a new sound: the cracking of enemy rifles firing directly at the approaching troops.

Chater stayed upright for a few more minutes, scrabbling to stand, desperately searching for shelter, and even managing to fire off a few rounds in the direction of the enemy. He could smell the battlefield as if it were a living thing, sweating cordite and blood, twisting and writhing as if trying to shake him off its back. His ears rang as bullets and shells burst close by, their jagged fragments ricocheting in all directions. One more step, and then another, and then an explosion, too close. A rag of hot metal slammed into his face, clawing its way through the soft flesh of his cheek and blasting away his teeth and the bones of his jaw.[7] As he rocked on his feet, absorbing the impact, a second fragment tore into his shoulder, bringing him crashing to the ground. Blood streamed into his eyes, blinding him, and the pain brought him to the edge of consciousness as his comrades pushed past him, continuing their desperate advance.

Chater remained where he had fallen, drifting in and out of the light, almost giving in to the darkness, when from somewhere he heard the shrill sound of an officer's whistle calling a halt to their advance. He could feel the pounding of heavy boots coming towards him, so he gathered up his last scraps of energy and managed to moan loudly enough to attract attention. He was hoisted up on strong arms and dragged away to the forward trenches. From there, the regiment's last remaining bearers managed to get him to the aid post in an abandoned farmhouse.[8] They laid him carefully down where the Regimental Medical Officer (RMO) would see him. They had little hope for the lad. Chater was drenched in blood, his face and shoulder ragged and filthy, and his breathing sounded as if all the debris of the town was stuck in his windpipe. The RMO had been treating the wounded of Neuve Chapelle all day and he was fighting to save every life he could.[9] He managed to slide a couple of morphine tablets into Chater's wreckage of a mouth, along with some splashes of water. Then, once the young man had calmed and his breathing had eased, he could gently dress his wounds, holding the pieces of his fractured face in place, easing open his clenched fists and murmuring something comforting that he hoped the soldier could hear. When he had done everything he could, the RMO called for bearers to take the stretcher to the next ambulance leaving for the hospital, sixty miles away up the Boulogne road.

In the ambulance, the morphine had begun to wear off as Chater drifted in and out of consciousness. Then there was another bump, but this time he heard the squeak of a handbrake and tyres crunching on gravel. The canvas flaps at the rear were folded back and he heard footsteps and voices, as the driver briefed the nurses and orderlies who had come to collect his load. Then the pain was back again, rolling in waves stronger than ever, as hurried hands jostled his stretcher out of the straps and into the open. He cried out as he was moved into the daylight, set down and then carried inside by two orderlies.

A nurse leaned over him, not able to see much past his blood-soaked bandages and matted hair, but knowing from his grey skin and his moans of agony that he was close to death. She had lost count of how many men she had escorted up the once-pristine flagstone steps of the hospital – 800 patients had arrived in just the thirty-six hours since the beginning of the battle, each one in a worse condition than the last.[10] At least Chater had seen a medical officer, if only for a minute or so; most men came in straight from the battlefield, covered in mud and dust, their wounds undressed, their blood dripping onto the floor of the ambulance or onto the man on the stretcher beneath. Sometimes ambulance drivers jumped down from their vehicles on arrival to warn orderlies and nurses that all had gone quiet in there a while back, so there was probably no hurry to unload. In one ambulance they had opened the doors to find a single survivor, trapped among the corpses of his comrades, having endured the sounds of their agony as they died one by one.[11]

Inside the hospital, the two bearers gently carried Chater on his stretcher as the nurse led them to the ward for the very worst cases. There was almost no room left and they had to carry him with the greatest care so as not to step on the stretchers lying between the beds, in the middle of the ward and out into the corridors. If Neuve Chapelle had been a victory, as everyone was saying, then the staff would hate to see a defeat. A doctor was brought to see Chater immediately and the nurse set to work removing his uniform and cleaning his face. She gently sponged away the blood that had caked one of his eyes shut. Chater blinked several times and then opened his eyes wide: no more blood splatters, just a white ceiling and the kind, tired face of a nurse drifting in and out of his vision. He was scheduled for surgery, she quietly explained. Nothing to worry about. He was safe now. As he finally fell asleep, he wondered at his war. Months of waiting and then just minutes of fighting. There would be no great victory for him to remember, only this pain. But also something else: the faces of all the men and women who had appeared before him, determined to fight for his life. Those were memories worth saving.

2

Bearers

Earnest Douglas, William Young, William Easton

> There was one thing I wanted to be, but feared I would not be
> equal to it. That was a stretcher bearer.
>
> William Young, March 1917

The call for bearer teams was the last thing a soldier heard in the
forward trenches before the final order to attack. 'Bearers up!'
were clear words in a human voice, echoing up and down the
line. Then everyone tried to look away as the Commanding Officer
(CO) checked his watch for the last time and reached for the
whistle around his neck. As the soldiers tried to distract themselves for the minutes or seconds remaining, they jostled the
bearer teams who were trying to squeeze in at the back of the
trench. They bumped up against the heavy wooden stretchers, as
if that would somehow charm them against being brought back
on one of them later. They yelled at the bearers to 'get a rifle' or
'do some fighting'.[1] Other soldiers turned their backs on the
bearers altogether, knowing what their presence meant and
blocking out the sight of the stretchers. The bearers themselves
stayed silent. They had done their talking back at the dugout,
when they checked on supplies, the final location of the aid posts
and exchanged addresses so that they knew who to write to, if
one of their team was killed.[2]

Then came the shriek of the whistles, sounding everywhere along
the line. Everyone turned to face forward. The soldiers panted and

roared, pushed themselves over the top and hurled themselves against the enemy. They shoved past the bearers, standing stock-still, waiting for the trench to empty. Then the bearers pushed the heavy stretchers out over the top and climbed the ladders, stepping onto the battlefield, slowly and silently, each keeping an eye on the others to make sure that the team stayed together. They pressed forward behind the men, straining to hear the first scream of agony amongst the roar of the attack. After the battle of Loos one bearer wrote home that it was very easy 'to do gallant deeds with arms in hands and when the blood is up but the courage demanded to walk quietly into a hail of lead to bandage and carry away a wounded man, that is worth talking about'.[3]

When Earnest Douglas joined the bearer corps he wanted to explain to his family what his job entailed and why he wasn't quite a soldier any longer. But he couldn't write to his parents directly because his mother couldn't stand the worry of seeing a letter with an army postmark. So instead Douglas sent his letters to their next-door neighbour, Gladys. Gladys would signal through her window that a letter had arrived, and his father would come and collect it and check its contents, before passing it on to his wife.

> Well, I'm a stretcher bearer. Whilst in the line . . . I've seen some very nasty sights and carried some nasty cases down, all under shell fire . . . Up past the knees in mud – balancing on the edge of shell craters, slipping and sliding, shells bursting above and in the earth all around us, it's God's mercy that we get through but we have the *patient* to think of and quickness probably means saving *his* life so we go right through it, not caring a damn and somehow – when you get to the sap-head and safety, you laugh and joke at all the capers we've been having and how 'that one' just missed us and so on . . . they talk about a soldier going out and fetching a comrade in under shell fire – and he gets the MM or DCM. *We* are always under shell fire and can't dump our *stretcher* and *run* for it to a safe spot, we have to *plod* on . . .

What annoys me most is when we get a chap 'serious' and make a dash and he dies at the door of the dressing place – love's labours lost. But I suppose it's God's will and he's 'the boss' . . . I am contented but if they gave me my ticket they wouldn't see my arse for dust in my rush for Blighty. If you hear anyone running a field ambulance down, tell 'em to allez and try it. I'm here Dad, and it's no good worrying.

Douglas hadn't become a stretcher bearer by default, as had been the case in the first few months of the war, when casualties had been dragged around the battlefield by bandsmen or pipers, or by anyone too big or too stupid to do proper soldiering. Douglas might have been unschooled, but he was bright and was immediately taken by the idea of the newly formed bearer corps when the Royal Army Medical Corps recruiter mentioned it to him. From the recruiter's point of view, Douglas fitted the official specifications perfectly: 'Stretcher bearers should be men of intelligence who are actually interested in their work, and on no account should they be men who have been selected because they are useless or physically incapable of regimental work.'[4]

Douglas had been particularly drawn to the training courses for the new stretcher-bearers corps. Like many of the men 'enlisting to apply the bandage', he felt that they were receiving a proper qualification that might come in handy after the war.[5] It didn't much feel like a proper qualification during the first four weeks of the course, though. Douglas needed to develop the physical strength and fitness required for bearing, so there were hours of marching up and down Box Hill in Surrey carrying a heavily weighted stretcher.[6] The tall ones in his class were always put on 'top-shelf duty', getting down stretchers from the top rack of the training ambulance. Several hours of that would do your back in. But, once they were strong enough, the course moved to the Army's own hospital, the Cambridge at Aldershot, where Douglas prepared to learn how to treat his patients as well as carry them.[7]

The course had its own textbook, *The Stretcher Bearer*, part of

the Oxford War Manuals series, rushed into print in early 1915.[8]
The book was well designed: small enough to fit into a tunic
pocket and full of photographs showing splints, slings and wound
dressings. It made things so clear that reading didn't even feel like
studying, and it made Douglas eager to get to the front. But then
came a taste of what he could expect in France. He was called
out at night to unload real casualties from hospital trains at
Aldershot station, and then used as a pall bearer for the funerals
of those patients that the Cambridge couldn't save.

The course lasted ten weeks and, when it had finished, Douglas
was sent across the Channel to the war itself. Some of his course-
mates had expressed concern that their new skills might not be
properly respected in France, but their supervisors told them not
to worry: the days when stretcher bearers were treated like
donkeys were over. Regimental medical officers had also been
getting some training. A new directive sent by the Royal Army
Medical Corps (RAMC) set it all out clearly:

> The RMO should always have the keenest regard for his own
> personnel of medical orderlies and the stretcher bearers. On the
> knowledge, initiative and courageous spirit of these men both he
> and the unit will have to rely greatly. Good orderlies and stretcher
> bearers are worth any amount of trouble. He should know them
> all by name, get to know their histories, should cultivate their
> acquaintance and understand their individual characteristics, so as
> to learn which of them is fit to be a leader in any undertaking
> . . . generally he should care for them in all ways to the very best
> of his powers.[9]

Not only would each bearer have the respect from his medical
colleagues that his skills deserved, explained the supervisor, but
his training would continue at the front line. The RMOs would
be giving a weekly lecture on medical subjects – a proper lecture,
not skipped or rushed.[10] Everyone, including the RMO, would go
on learning.

And so it was when Douglas got to France. Once a week, provided they weren't needed out on the battlefield, Douglas's medical officer gathered his bearers around him in his dugout and told them to start a new page in their notebooks. The heading for one of the very first lectures Douglas heard was 'PANNIER'. Panniers were used to carry a bearer's supplies. They were made either of wicker, like fishing creels, or canvas, like satchels, with a red cross painted on the side. Every bearer was responsible for his own pannier and for the supplies inside it. If they lost an item, they had to make sure they went and got a replacement before going back out for casualties. Scissors, for instance, were lost as easily on the battlefield as lives, slipping out of cold hands down into the mud, never to be seen again. But scissors were essential. You needed them to trim dressings to size and to cut through uniforms so that you could get to the wounds.

Douglas learned he should always check that his water bottle was full and, if there was room, take a spare. Wounded men were often badly dehydrated and gulped down a bottle's worth in one go. In a little square tin there were blue morphine tablets. If the casualty couldn't swallow them on his own, you could slide the tablet under his tongue and let it dissolve. But you had to remember how much morphine you'd given him or there could be a problem later on. Make sure you take your crayon to make a note, or write on his forehead so that the medics at the aid post can immediately see if he's had a dose. And stuff dressings into every spare inch of the pannier. Dressings weren't only used on simple wounds, but were crucial to the control of haemorrhage, as they'd called it back at the Cambridge – Stopping the bleeding, in other words. Take a big handful of dressings and press them down on the bleed, and keep pressing down until it stopped or you got to the aid post. Tourniquets were only to be used as a last resort. Leave a tourniquet on too long and a limb could be lost. But let a patient bleed too long and a life could be lost. How to stop a bleed was perhaps the most important thing Douglas had learned on his course. If you couldn't stop a bleed, there wasn't much point even coming to France.

It was several months before Douglas went home on leave, and when he did his mother grasped his hands and wept at the state of them. Everyone at the front could spot a bearer by his hands. The wooden handles of the stretchers quickly started to deteriorate. They got shot at, or had bits broken off, and the splinters were the very devil. In the wet the wood rotted, splitting the handle ends. All that bearers could do was wind a length of wire round the handles to keep them together, but the wire would cut their hands to pieces. Gloves weren't much help. They made it difficult to get a grip on the wood, and no one ever kept a pair of gloves for very long at the front. Douglas had bearer's hands: a mix of blisters and calluses, first rubbed raw and then scar-cracked and worn.

He couldn't hide his hands, but during the rest of his leave Douglas took care not to take off his shirt in front of his parents. His back and shoulders were in an even worse state. His patients were often dead weights – he had trained with a twelve-stone weight, but he often had to carry more, plus blankets. And although the official bearer complement was six, there were rarely enough men available, so two or three were more usual. The load was concentrated all on one shoulder under a wide leather halter strap, crossed over the head. The strap bit down through tunic or greatcoat, and gradually the ache turned to a burn, as the flesh rubbed raw and the muscles and joints strained. Bearers folded up sandbags and put them under the straps, but after a while – and especially in the wet – these didn't make much difference. Slowly the strap would slide off the shoulder and down onto the neck, and a bearer would gasp out that he was choking and they would all stop. Then the straps were taken off and the sandbags rearranged, and after a few deep breaths they would continue.[11] If they were lucky they managed to travel another 200 yards or so before having to stop again. Even the shortest trips could take hours.

After his mother had cried herself to sleep after his first day back home, Douglas sat up with his father and tried to answer his questions. Most of what he did was 'the carry' – getting a casualty on their stretcher to the aid post. There were hardly any easy carries. Night carries were probably the safest. Both sides had their bearers out then, and their sanitary squads were collecting the dead, so mostly you didn't get shot at. But you still didn't flaunt yourself. Sometimes Douglas carried a torch – if the batteries had stayed dry – and flashed it on and off so that the team could see where they were going, but they still tripped over corpses or duckboards and got tangled up in barbed wire. Sometimes they simply got lost and lumbered about for hours, looking for familiar landmarks.[12] And the night-time battlefield had its own lullaby, with bearers calling out and listening for any response. Back and forth, back and forth they called, not too loudly, to avoid alerting the enemy, but hopefully loud enough for those trapped in shell holes to hear them; then they fell silent, straining to catch any reply. When they finally got back into the trenches, they found that the soldiers there had been listening – their lullaby had not sent them to sleep, but kept them awake, in fear for their fallen comrades.[13]

But when Douglas came to think about it, the one thing that really affected them badly was the weather. If it was warm, they had to take off their coats and then their backs really got a mangling.[14] Sweat dripped into their eyes, making it difficult to see where they were going – and when they rubbed their eyes with their muddy hands, they cursed that now they couldn't see anything at all. But then cold weather wasn't any better. Cold froze the ground and made it slippery. It numbed their hands and feet. And cold often killed a patient before they could get him to the aid post.

By far the worst was the rain. It saturated their clothes – an army greatcoat could absorb seven or eight pounds of water on its own – and those of their patients, as well as any blankets or bandages. Wet leather straps stiffened and rubbed more than ever. Wet hands slipped on wet stretcher handles. Worst of all, rain turned the battlefield into mud, threatening to suck you down to your doom. The bearers put layers of empty sandbags over their boots to give them extra grip in the mud – one soldier said he looked like a stage elephant going out in layers of grey folds – but that too was of little use.

In deep mud after heavy rain one of the team had to lead the way so that they wouldn't fall or become trapped. Some shell holes were big enough to bury a bus in and, when they got wet, their edges could easily subside. If one of the bearers slipped and fell, he could drag everyone down to the bottom. Then they had to gather themselves, disentangle the stretcher straps, reload the patient and crawl out again. Douglas had to focus hard on listening to the leader call each step on their journey. It took a huge effort to remain calm while you crawled along like a big muddy tortoise.[15] What he didn't tell his father was that stopping could mean death. At Arras, one entire team and their patient were killed after they became stuck in the mud and were blown to pieces by enemy shelling – the last bearer falling over the stretcher as if to protect the man they had been carrying.[16]

But stretcher bearers didn't always mind the rain. If there were no carries, they went outside and held up their faces and their callused hands so that the rain could wash away the grime.

William Young was a soldier in the Post Office Rifles when he made his first carry. One day, out on the battlefield after the fighting had stopped, he had found a mate badly wounded in the stomach. He ran back to the aid post, but there were no bearers left. The harassed Medical Officer (MO) gave him some dressings and a water bottle and told him what to do for the casualty. Young did his best, but realised that the man was too heavy for him to move on his own. So he stayed with him, waving and calling out for help until he attracted the attention of some soldiers. Together they loaded up the man and carried him to the aid post. Young was transformed by the experience: he had saved one life among so much death. After his first period of service was over, he immediately re-enlisted in the RAMC and, after some time in the training trenches at Étaples, was transferred to a Field Ambulance for the second Line Battalion, 174th Brigade.[17]

One of his first jobs was to bring back a wounded man lying in a deep shell hole. When Young ran over, he was spotted by an enemy sniper, who began to fire at him. It was now too dangerous for his teammates to join him, so Young stayed in the hole with the casualty, with the sniper pinning him down for hours, firing every time he moved.[18] All Young could do for the man was slowly turn his head so that he faced him, and hold his hand. He whispered a few words, told the soldier his name and that everything would be all right: eventually the bloody sniper would get bored and move on. He tried to smile, but he wasn't sure the man could see his expression through the mud on his face. When he saw that the soldier was crying, Young squeezed his hand and tried to comfort him. The soldier shook his head almost imperceptibly and then looked away. It wasn't the pain, he whispered. He was so sorry – he didn't deserve to be saved. He'd been one of those who had ridiculed the bearers while they waited to go over the top. The man was sobbing openly now, and Young was worried about the sniper hearing them. He shushed the wounded man firmly. It didn't matter any more, he whispered – the bearers understood.

Finally the soldier calmed, but the sniper had heard him and started firing again. The men lay together in fear and silence for what felt like hours, the bearer holding his patient's hand. Then the sound of the shots drifted away. The sniper had found another target. Carefully Young got up onto his elbows and started dressing the soldier's wounds, giving him water and morphine. He now saw that the man was small and light, so he could probably carry him on his own. By now it was dark and it was getting cold. Young felt he couldn't wait any longer. Hoisting the patient up onto his back, he climbed out of the crater. When the sniper saw them and began firing, it was too late to go back, so Young ran for their lives. Shots followed him all the way back to the British lines, but he ducked and weaved and managed to keep them both safe. At the aid post, he laid the soldier down and re-dressed his wounds. He had spent so much time with him, in such danger, that he was reluctant to let him go. Most bearers felt like that about their patients, particularly after a long carry. As one bearer put it, sometimes their going was like that of an old friend, who shared the rigours of the journey.[19]

But Young's war as a bearer really began in April 1917 at Bullecourt during the battle of Arras, where thousands of wounded men lay abandoned on the great, bloody Douai plain. His team arrived in the evening and were setting up their post when a group of soldiers ran up. Their mates were trapped in a shell hole, they told the bearers, all of them badly hurt. They had to find them, quickly. One of the soldiers tried to show them on a map where the wounded men were, but Bullecourt had been completely destroyed and Young and the team spent hours stumbling over barbed wire and mud, constantly under enemy fire, having to find their way. When they finally reached the spot the soldier had marked on the map, no one was there, alive or dead. So they struggled back and it took them two hours in the dark and cold to reach their trenches.

Young didn't know what was worse: not finding any casualties or not being able to get to them. One of the bearers had been at Mametz Wood the previous year, where they had been pinned down in shell holes and trenches and all they could do was listen to the screaming of the wounded. They hadn't expected to survive, let alone get to the men. But when the fighting stopped they found that their troubles had only just started. The wood was full of smashed, upturned trees and deep troughs and ditches, which made it impossible to use a stretcher. Every single casualty had to be brought out on someone's back, in the dark. The bearers stumbled and fell for hours, cursing and apologising to the wounded, many of whom bled to death as they carried them.[20]

Young didn't sleep much for the remainder of his first night at Bullecourt. He had been a soldier and, if you reported the location of wounded comrades, you usually didn't get it wrong. As soon as it was light he would go out again. His teammates had been given other carries, so he found some volunteers from the wounded men's regiment and loaded them up with panniers and

stretchers. They got permission from the officers, on condition
that the chaplain said a special blessing over them. It didn't bode
well, but out they went, under heavy enemy shelling – and the
chaplain's blessing seemed to work. Young and the volunteers
found the shell hole and the twelve casualties lying at its bottom.

Young thought he had never seen anything worse. The wounded
had been abandoned for days and were dehydrated, gangrenous
and paralysed with fear. He began to dress their wounds and give
out morphine and water, instructing his volunteers to follow his
example. Even Young's expert handling caused them to cry out
in pain, never mind the fumblings of the soldiers. But Young kept
steady, reassuring the wounded men: they'd all soon be in a nice
warm hospital bed or back in Blighty, not to worry. But all the
while he knew that many would end up on the amputation table
or in the moribund ward.

Finally they were ready to move. Young's best friend in the
bearer team, George, had found his way to the shell hole in search
of his comrade. The two bearers now showed the volunteers how
best to move the men onto stretchers and, one by one, they sent
them back through an old trench network to avoid enemy shells.
When Young turned to pick up the last casualty he found that
they were one stretcher short. The soldier was just a boy and his
leg was almost gone, so Young hoisted him up onto his back and
carried him down himself, alternating with George. The old trench
network was collapsing and the men were struggling to make
their way through it, so whichever bearer wasn't carrying led the
way. The last part of the carry was over open ground, and shells
slammed into the earth around them as soon as they left the
trenches. But somehow they made it. The colonel and the chaplain were astounded. After being summoned to the adjutant's tent
for cocoa – it was all he had to offer them at that moment – Young
and George returned to their tent at the field ambulance, where
they talked about their day for a good while.

At Passchendaele, Young was leading a team of bearers and
thirty walking wounded when a shell struck the group, killing

several bearers and their casualties, and injuring many more. Young kept his nerve and managed to lead the survivors into a nearby pillbox. It wasn't much, but it was safe from shelling. The men had few stores, very little water, and some of the wounded had begun to cry that the enemy would find them, throw in a grenade and they would all be killed. All night the bearers treated the severely wounded men, rationing the water, cutting the dressings into ever smaller patches. As the pillbox gradually grew quiet, Young found himself looking after a big, strong man who had lost half his head. Young sat by his side, trying to calm the raging soldier who struggled to get up and leave until the moment he died. When the water finally ran out, they had to leave the pillbox. Outside, the enemy guns had presumed them dead and moved on. But the danger wasn't over. The ground was liquid mud and the bearers had to wade their way back to their lines, stretchers held high. It took them three trips, but everyone made it. There wasn't an aid post where Young expected to find it and no doctor either, so he set up his own post and treated the men for three more days until he was relieved.

On quiet evenings the bearers gathered together in one of their tents. Often they talked while mending their uniforms, which had been torn when the men they were carrying clawed at them in agony. One of them had a sewing kit and another a little tin of buttons, which he passed round. This was a time to think back, to make sense, to try and mend – not just their tunics, but themselves.

Everyone had a story of madness to tell. One of them had recently been at an aid post where a bearer team had just returned, covered in blood (and worse) literally up to their waists. It turned out they'd been carrying all night, and at dawn they had got back to the head of a communication trench crowded with soldiers waiting for the whistle. The leading bearer dropped down into the trench and waited for them to move. None of them did. Bloody infantry, he thought. His team was still up there, becoming a target, as the offensive was about to begin. He gave the usual call of 'Gangway stretcher bearers!' Everyone normally moved for the gangway call, for it meant that a wounded man was on board. It had no effect. He tried again: 'Make way for wounded!' Still nothing. When he walked over and pushed at the shoulder of one of the men leaning on the trench wall, the soldier's head lolled back. He was dead. It turned out that every last one of them was dead, hit where they stood, the trench too crowded for anyone to have fallen back. The shelling was heavy and they had no choice but to use the trench; leaving the stretcher on top, they started to push the dead soldiers over. Then they got the stretcher down and told the casualty to keep his eyes shut and not to open them, whatever happened. They set off over the human mound, two of them dragging the stretcher behind them, the other two up ahead, pushing over the corpses to make a path. They kept tripping up, their legs squishing down into the soft corpses, but they carried on and returned covered in blood.[21]

At least corpses were quiet. If most bearers thought about it, they probably preferred a trench full of dead soldiers to living ones. They all hated arriving with a casualty at the top of a forward trench full of excited, adrenalin-fuelled soldiers, ready for the attack. When they dropped down into a trench with the torn-up patient on their stretcher, there was usually a stunned silence. The bearers could sense the men's excitement draining away and hear stifled sobs of fear.[22] So they kept their heads down and hurried as best they could. But then bearers were probably, the maddest of them all. Look at us, said one of the battle-hardened team leaders: sitting here in a tent, sewing on buttons like old maids, with the toe of a boot on a German corpse sticking up through the floor and all of us pretending not to notice.

William Easton of the 77th Field Ambulance often thought about how much he had learned since he became a stretcher bearer. 'INOCULATIONS' was one important lesson. The MO had taught him how to give injections, and now his team went around inoculating whole battalions against typhoid. 'FEET' would have been another heading in his notebook. Bearers spent hours rubbing frozen soles and toes to keep away frostbite and trench foot, and watched out for marching injuries such as sores, blisters and damaged tendons.[23] 'MORPHINE' was a section they kept adding to as they grew more experienced as bearers. In the beginning they had all doled out the blue morphine tablets to anyone who so much as groaned, but as they came to understand the carry, they tried not to give out so much. An unconscious patient was a dead weight; patients who were awake were lighter and could tell you what hurt and if they were suddenly beginning to bleed. Moreover, giving out morphine on the carry meant there was less available for patients at the aid post. So, like most bearers, Easton had become good at negotiating with wounded men who begged for morphine; sometimes just calm confidence had the same sort of effect.[24]

Bearers understood the weight of a casualty better than anyone. If you ran out of stretchers, you shouldn't use a greatcoat or a blanket to fetch someone in. Everyone made that mistake in the early days, but the patients got too bumped in a bundle, their wounds opened up again and it was much more effort than it looked. Instead you should take them on your back. You could get further than you thought, once the patient was hoisted up, and the weight of him kept you going somehow.

Then there was 'GAS'. In 1916 the bearers' training course was expanded to include time at 'Gas School'. Easton was one of those who had learned about the effects of gas, how to carry a gas mask, and how to get a mask on a patient whilst he tried to wrench it off. His notebook might also have included a page headed 'AID POST'. It wasn't just a question of dumping down your stretcher when you got there. Sometimes the MO was busy, or even dead, so it was up to the bearer to keep the post going. On arrival the bearer would often fill out a Field Medical Card (called a 'ticket'), cut a patient's hair away from a head wound and trim back tunic rags. He would try to keep his patient alive until the MO or the ambulance came, and would then give them details of his wounds and what he had done for him. Working in the aid post always made Easton want to learn more about medicine. There was a Canadian bearer team that had assembled a small library containing first-aid and medical textbooks sent by one of their wives.[25] Easton, like many bearers by 1917, could take a parade of the sick and run an aid post, if there was no MO to do it.

But there were other things he had learned that didn't make it into his notebook. German, for starters. Bearers often had to supervise groups of POWs to help with carries to the rear.[26] Sometimes you even had a POW as a patient on your own carry. Either way, it helped to know a bit of pidgin German, but Easton didn't think it would be sensible to write down his vocab in his notebook. You never knew who might get the wrong idea. Quite often they came across German medical supplies and discovered that they were much better than their own. German bearers had big absorbent pads for wounds and sticky tape to fasten them with – much more efficient than the thin cotton wads with tails that Easton had to use. Any time you found German supplies, you kept them, although as the war went on, you had to be careful. Sometimes the retreating Germans left behind a cache of supplies that was booby-trapped. One of the bearer teams kept a fishing rod so that they could prod desirable items, such as binoculars, from a distance, to be sure they were safe.[27]

Then there were the things he had learned about on the battle-field itself. After two years of war the trench networks were beginning to crumble and collapse. But new trenches weren't always built with the bearer in mind. They were so deep and narrow that, once you got down in them, it could suddenly be very dark except for the strip of sky above.[28] They had sharp angles and corners where you had to lift the stretcher up high to pass through. Some of them weren't more than two feet wide, and a queue of bearers could build up on top waiting for a space to lower their carry – and a queue of bearers drew snipers. Easton didn't really care much for the new style of trench. Those wretched engineers dug them so quickly that it was easy to get lost in a labyrinth of new routes. Then you had to go back up and try and get your bearings – without getting shot – and remember the changes so that you could put them on your map.

'MAPS' – a single sheet of paper, but so important. Medical officers or senior bearers had to be good at drawing. New maps were issued just before the beginning of an offensive, and whole evenings were spent poring over them, crayons in hand, adding new trenches or erasing collapsed ones. Bearers wrapped their maps in a small piece of oilskin cloth to keep them dry.

Easton could have thought of other lectures to add to the stretcher-bearer syllabus. One of them would be about 'WALKING WOUNDED'. Bearer parties attracted long lines of lightly wounded men who followed them, knowing they would lead them to the nearest aid post. Yet lines of bandaged men also attracted enemy fire, so bearers had to learn to keep the group together and out of sight. They also had to be inventive when it came to organising 'TRANSPORT'. One team fully loaded with stretchers, and with many walking wounded behind them, came across a working party of twenty Scottish soldiers who were digging a roadside ditch.[29] The bearers persuaded them to stop their work and use their wheelbarrows to carry those on the point of collapse.

'SLEEP'. A bearer should sleep whenever he could. He should be able to sleep in spite of the sound of guns thump-thumping all night long. He should also ignore the smell of decomposing human flesh: it was the exhalation of the battlefield.[30] One bearer returning from forty-six hours of continuous duty at the second battle of Ypres simply dropped to the floor of his billet and went instantly to sleep as the battle raged around him. Sometimes Easton could only snatch a few minutes here and there on a stretcher at a medical post or casualty clearing station (CCS). The nurses carefully stepped over him because they knew how much he needed the rest.

'FOOD': bearers should eat whatever, and whenever, they could and should learn to scavenge. Rations were often late and small, so during any lull in the fighting bearers should look for food on the bodies of the dead. A corpse had no use for a tin of bully beef, and sometimes you came upon abandoned rations and stores.[31] One of Easton's friends, who had been a bearer at Loos, still talked about the magnificent meal conjured up by one of the men in his battalion, who had managed to brew up some tea, make some toast and bacon and even find a slice of sultana cake. Bearers should never go hungry. Ask your family to send food, and use your own wages to buy extra. A younger member of a team of bearers seemed to grow an inch every month, so whilst most of his colleagues spent their money on beer and brandy, he bought himself supplies of chocolate, bread and eggs. He too would rather have had the beer, but life as a stretcher bearer gave him a tremendous appetite.[32]

Perhaps the last lecture ought to be on 'ANIMALS', with a subsection on 'MOLES'. There was no defeating a mole. One bearer team was trying to get some sleep in a new dugout, but was woken by clods of earth landing on their faces. It was a company of moles digging their route away from the battlefield. For several nights the bearers bayoneted the area, but the guns kept firing and the moles kept coming, so eventually they gave up and moved to a different dugout.

'PETS' were better company. If the team was based in one place for a while, it should think about getting a pet, preferably a dog. There were plenty of dogs roaming the battlefield, abandoned by their owners. Having a pet gave you something to look after that wasn't a broken man. And pets were funny. One team, on an easy carry, came across a small puppy that was about to drown in a flooded shell hole. One of the bearers found his way to the bottom and rescued the dog. They wrapped him in a tunic and stowed him between the boots of the casualty they were carrying. Back at the aid post, they used a mountain of dressings and blanket rags to clean him up. A neat white terrier was revealed beneath the sludge, which responded quickly to his treatment of tinned sardines and small pieces of chocolate, so the team decided to keep him. But when the tent flap was opened unexpectedly the dog ran out and flung himself in the nearest puddle, rolling around in the mud until not a trace of white fur could be seen. It seemed that the puppy had also learned how to survive on the Western Front. 'These men,' complained one medical officer of his bearers, 'will keep pets under any circumstances.'[33]

There was plenty of hard work that needed doing when the bearers weren't out on the field. They mended broken trenches and dug aid posts. They hollowed out resting places in trenches along their communication routes, so that they had somewhere to safely stow a casualty during a long carry. If they remembered a particularly tricky length of trench that needed widening, they did it themselves.[34] They left caches of stretchers and blankets in forward dugouts, to have them readily available when the attack came.[35] And they found wood and built tables and benches to furnish new aid posts. It was hard work, for sure, but bearers never really minded the grind of repair and rebuilding. It kept them busy and fit for the carries to come.[36]

Easton needed all his resources, physical and mental, when he travelled on the Menin Road in September 1917. Sappers had hung tarpaulins between the trees along one section of the road, to screen the bearer teams who were going back and forth to a small aid post in a cottage that was filling with casualties. But when the enemy spotted and shelled the place, everyone was killed. Easton's team found itself trapped on the blood-drenched road, the men flinging themselves into a ditch to protect themselves and their casualties.

When the enemy fire finally died away, Easton headed for another aid post located in an elephant dugout, a metallic prefab thought to be the safest form of shelter on the front. He left his casualties there and went back for more wounded from the field. When he returned he found that a shell had hit the dugout, penetrating its metal walls and ricocheting around the structure, killing everyone inside. Easton sat with his casualty and waited until the sanitary squad arrived. He tried not to watch them as they cleaned out the shelter, but he couldn't help overhearing that they had been told to bring sandbags rather than blanket coffins, as everyone inside had been cut to pieces. After that, Easton would never touch another sandbag, no matter how blistered his shoulder or how muddy his boots.

Bearers learned more about death than any other men on the battlefield. They learned how to read the iron voices of the guns, how to hear them shout their power and know what sacrifices they required that day.[37] They learned not to fear death, as it followed them on each carry. They learned to recognise its work, to see instantly who was dead and who was still alive. They learned to watch men die. They learned how to help them out of this world, either with soft words or with a strong dose of morphine.[38] They learned how to turn away from the dying and find others who would live. It was never easy. One bearer left a man to die because others needed him more. But it troubled him all day, so in the evening he went back, found that the man was alive and fetched him in.[39] He never found out if the soldier survived, but at least he was able to sleep. Bearers also got used to the seriously wounded men who waved them away, sending them to more deserving cases nearby. And they always made sure there were matches and cigarettes in their panniers, kept dry in their oilskin alongside their map, so that they could give a dying man a last smoke.

They learned not to mind the long, desperate carry that ended with the casualty going straight to the moribund ward, where a chaplain waited for him, rather than a surgeon, or those they delivered straight to the sanitary squads for burial. Sometimes it helped them to keep little memories of the men they hadn't been able to save, like a bloodstained paybook or a button pressed into their hand as a parting gift.[40] They got used to getting up on mornings when their first task was to check on the casualties laid outside the aid post and remove the dead from stretchers that were needed by the living.[41] And they learned about death among their own: sometimes they would need to build new teams when the old one had been utterly destroyed.[42] They learned not to get annoyed when a new back wasn't as broad or as strong as that of an old comrade. The new arrival would soon learn; his hands would toughen, and the carry would go on.

One of the chaplains at the front marvelled at the determination and courage of the bearer teams around him. He watched them closely, often going out on the carry with them, and he listened as they spoke to their casualty along the way. He noticed the little phrases they repeated over and over again as they went about their work, and one day he wrote them down and found that together they made a poem:

> Easy does it – a bit o' trench 'ere,
> Mind that blinkin' bit o' wire,
> There's a shell 'ole on your left there,
> Lift 'im up a little 'igher.
> Stick it, lad, ye'll soon be there now,
> Want to rest 'ere for a while?
> Let 'im dahn then – gently – gently,
> There ye are, lad. That's the style.
> Want a drink, mate? 'Ere's my bottle,
> Lift 'is 'ead up for 'im, Jack,
> Put my tunic underneath 'im
> 'Ow's that, chummy? That's the tack!
> Guess we'd better make a start now,
> Ready for another spell?
> Best be goin', we won't 'urt ye,
> But 'e might just start to shell.
> Are ye right, mate? Off we goes then.
> That's well over on the right,
> Gawd Almighty, that's a near un!
> 'Old your end up good and tight.
> Never mind, lad, you're for Blighty,
> Mind this rotten bit o' board.

We'll soon 'ave ye tucked in bed, lad
'Opes ye gets to my old ward.
No more war for you, my 'earty,
This'll get ye well away,
Twelve good months in dear old Blighty,
Twelve good months if you're a day,
MO's got a bit o' something
What'll stop that blarsted pain.
'Ere's a rotten bit o' ground, mate,
Lift up 'igher – up again,
Wish 'e'd stop 'is blarsted shellin'
Makes it rotten for the lad.
When a feller's been and got it,
It affec's 'im twice as bad.
'Ow's it goin' now then, sonny?
'Ere's that narrow bit o' trench,
Careful, mate, there's some dead Jerries,
Lawd Almighty, what a stench!
'Ere we are now, stretcher-case, boys,
Bring him aht a cup o' tea!
Inasmuch as ye have done it
Ye have done it unto Me.[43]

3

Regimental Medical Officers

John Linnell, William Kelsey Fry,
Geoffrey Hardwick, Charles McKerrow

It seems to take a vast amount of firing to kill a man.

Charles McKerrow, 14 September 1915

Neuve Chapelle provided RMO John Linnell with the memory that would stay with him for the rest of his life. On the second day of the battle he had led the 23rd Field Ambulance attached to the Grenadier Guards to an aid post in an abandoned farmhouse. There had barely been time to explore the sturdy old building – although he discovered, to his delight, that it had a working tap – before the courtyard and stable block filled with stretchers and walking wounded. Linnell and his team worked for several hours without stopping, the bearers bringing them one grimy, battered, terrified man after another (one of them was Mickey Chater). Eventually they blurred into one bloody line as the medics dressed wounds, gave out morphine and ordered men into ambulances to take them to the base hospitals.

Then, at a time when Linnell was beginning to feel unable to cope with the sheer number of arrivals for much longer, a young gunnery officer wandered in. It was all right, he told the RMO so quietly that Linnell had to lean forward to hear him. He didn't need much, he said, but he had received a biff in the back, so he would sit down for a moment, if the doc wouldn't mind. There was something about him – a distracted calmness – so Linnell didn't call over a bearer, but helped the man sit down on a bit of wall. The young officer sighed and looked off into the distance. He made no protest when Linnell lifted up his tunic to examine his back. A piece of shell fragment had blown a hole in him, front to back. When Linnell squatted down to get a better look, he could see all the way through the young man to the fields beyond. When he got to his feet, the officer got up too. He stood still, breathing quietly. Linnell pressed some morphine tablets into his hand, gave him a water canteen and watched as the man walked out of the farmhouse.

Linnell struggled not to let this one patient overwhelm him. He had other problems. Word had got out about the aid post and now cavalry troops, motor carriers, stray soldiers as well as an endless stream of casualties were heading to the farmhouse from all over the battlefield to shelter behind its thick walls. Soon they were becoming a target themselves. Three shells hit the exterior walls and, with every explosion, the gun aimers got closer and closer. Linnell realised that they were trapped. They would have to stay in the farmhouse, even though the bombardment was getting so heavy that many of the casualties thought they were back on the battlefield.

So they worked on in the courtyard and stables, half-blinded by brick dust, dashing from shelter to shelter to avoid the shrapnel. The main dressing room received a direct hit, killing a German POW and further wounding the men being bandaged, but somehow missing their doctors. A huge piece of shrapnel quivered in the plaster over their heads, but they worked on. More and more holes appeared in the walls and ceiling. The patients waiting to be evacuated watched the debris of trees and buildings flying up into the sky, then crashing down around them. Suddenly one of them spotted a Royal Flying Corps (RFC) aircraft. The pilot flew his machine in wild loops, drawing the enemy fire away from the farmhouse, and everyone stopped to watch and cheer. Then they heard clattering hooves and squealing metal wheels as several horse-drawn guns arrived, the drivers shouting like madmen and flogging the horses on. The battery positioned itself just below the farmhouse and opened fire on the enemy guns that had shelled the farmhouse. Within minutes the German position fell silent.

Most of Linnell's patients could now be moved on. Darkness came and the little farmhouse grew quiet as the doctors and their remaining patients fell asleep on stretchers or fragments of wall, all feeling safer for the presence of the gun crews outside, watching over them. In the morning, after a short church service from the regimental chaplain, the work began again: guns and wounded, over and over, all day. In the evening, as the fighting slowed for the very last time, Linnell looked up to see a little queue of ambulances and trucks outside the aid post, waiting to take them all away. As he loaded up the last truck with their remaining supplies, he looked back at what remained of the farmhouse. There, just outside the walls, he saw the body of the young gunnery officer. He lay where he had fallen, only a few steps away from the wall where Linnell had examined him the day before.

William Kelsey Fry and his bearer teams of the 7th Division Royal Welch Fusiliers had made it safely out of Neuve Chapelle and joined their battalion in the first Artois offensive of May 1915. By then they had already gained a reputation as one of the best medical teams at the front. Frank Pearce and George Sheasby were Kelsey Fry's bearer team leaders, and the Fusiliers got used to seeing the three men together, pointing out features on the battlefield and conferring about conditions – doc and bearers indistinguishable one from the other.

On 9 May, the Fusiliers were ordered to take a small town close to the Aubers Ridge. It took them three days to conquer Festubert's sad streets, lined with ruined houses and charred tree stubs, and they suffered their heaviest casualty load of the war so far. The bearer teams were quickly overwhelmed by the numbers of wounded, and Kelsey Fry himself went out onto the battlefield to retrieve casualties. Time after time he cleaned the mud off his glasses, braced himself and joined the fighting soldiers, oblivious to all but the cries of the man he was trying to find in the middle of the chaos. When he found him, Kelsey Fry hoisted him up onto his back and ran as fast as he could. During one of these trips he was shot in both legs. The wounds weren't serious, but he was losing blood and lucky to make it back to the medical post with his patient. His bravery earned him a Military Cross (MC) for conspicuous gallantry and devotion to duty whilst under heavy fire.[1] His leg wounds earned him a short spell in hospital.

The division was sent to join a second assault on the Aubers Ridge in September 1915 at the battle of Loos, where chlorine gas was used for the first time. British tactics were completely inept. Men were ordered to advance straight towards heavily defended German trenches, bristling with machine guns. So many were killed that when the troops finally turned to retreat, the German gunners, repelled by the slaughter, ceased firing. The enemy even sent out their own medical personnel to help bearers like Frank Pearce who were trying to bring in some of the 8,000 casualties.[2] Loos earned Pearce a Distinguished Conduct Medal (DCM) for his bravery from 25 to 29 September, when he carried wounded men from the field on his back for forty-eight hours without stopping.[3]

In between battles, Kelsey Fry got on with the mundane duties of an RMO. If there was no fighting, much of his day was spent on sanitary work.[4] Every time the battalion moved, it was his responsibility to find a fresh-water supply and to make sure it didn't get polluted. This was a task that could take up days of his time. Once rivers were found, the water had to be tested as being fresh. If there was no river, wells were dug down to a water source. Then holes for 200-gallon water tanks had to be dug and filled – and hopefully he hadn't run out of chlorine supplies. And then there were the latrines: Kelsey Fry had to site, dig and maintain them. No wonder some RMOs complained that their work could be dull.[5]

The RMO also had to keep his men as clean as possible, which meant regular inspections of their kitbags, enamel mugs and feet; enamel mugs were standard issue at the front – they didn't smash and were easily cleaned. Some RMOs made their men feel like criminals, but not Kelsey Fry. He had this smile, the men of the Welch Fusiliers all agreed, that somehow made a difference. Men who had only met him once, being brought to him on a stretcher, felt the same. They listened to his calm and reassuring voice as he inspected their wounds, tore out a Field Medical Card from the large book they came in and fastened it to their tunic.[6] His voice alone could make you feel better and quieten your mind.[7] Not that he was soft. Everyone knew about his courage under fire and he exercised real authority. There were few officers at the front who could make men move quite as quickly as William Kelsey Fry.[8]

By 1916, the 'Year of Battles', Kelsey Fry's reputation had reached the upper ranks of the RAMC. They decided to promote him away from the dirt and gunfire of the front line to a safer post, heading one of the new casualty clearing stations, but Kelsey Fry refused. He felt that he could not serve his country as well there as he could at the front. In March the Welch Fusiliers were sent to Verdun, and now it was George Sheasby's turn to get a DCM for his bravery.[9] When orders came to prepare for a new offensive in the early summer, Kelsey Fry was told to oversee the creation of an entirely new aid post and several new teams of bearers. No one knew the date of the offensive, but their post was to be up and running as soon as possible so that it could receive the soldiers who were wounded going out into no-man's-land after dark to prepare the battlefield.

One of the aid post's very first patients was the poet Siegfried Sassoon. He had been cutting enemy wire at night when he was shot by a sniper. His injuries were not life-threatening, but he confessed to Kelsey Fry at the aid post that he hoped they might earn him an MC. Sassoon was moved to a casualty clearing station, which Kelsey Fry was visiting when the news came through that he had indeed won his medal. Knowing how much it meant to the young soldier, Kelsey Fry hurried over to the ward to tell him. Seeing that Sassoon was visibly disappointed not to have received the actual decoration right away, Kelsey Fry went to find a nurse to ask for a needle and thread. Then he sat down on Sassoon's bed, took off his tunic and unpicked his own faded medal ribbon, hard won at Festubert. He sewed it carefully onto Sassoon's tunic and handed it to the young soldier, with a smile. Sassoon always kept the doctor's ribbon, even though he would eventually reject his own medal.[10]

Sassoon missed the early months of the Somme as it took longer for him to recover from his injury than he would have liked. His comrades in the Welch Fusiliers kept him posted with regular letters telling him of their rough time, when they had lost 200 men in just three days. Kelsey Fry, Pearce and Sheasby didn't have time to write letters. They worked for two months straight, moving from medical post to medical post as the offensive bucked and surged, with the casualty load never slowing. At the end of August they found themselves at Guillemont Wood, where British and German forces fought each other fruitlessly in preparation for another, larger offensive in early September. There was hardly time to prepare a medical post, so they simply dug a hole as deep as time and the enemy would allow and put a tarpaulin over it. It filled with casualties almost immediately, like rain collecting in a puddle. As at every aid post on the line, they worked so hard that they stopped hearing the shellfire and didn't notice as it crept closer and closer.

The first Sassoon heard of the tragedy was when he received a letter in hospital.[11] At four o'clock on 29 August a shell had hit Kelsey Fry's medical post and exploded. Everyone knew the doctor and his team were in the post at the time, along with five severely wounded men, and, despite continuing shellfire, ran to help. But it was too late: Pearce and Sheasby had both been killed, along with all their patients and two other bearers. Under unremitting fire, the soldiers and orderlies dug and dug, pulling out body after body until they found their doctor – miraculously alive among the death and debris – covered in the blood of his closest comrades. The man who had carried so many casualties from the battlefield was now carried away himself, his bright eyes closed and his smile gone. Kelsey Fry would survive, but never recovered sufficiently to return to the front. For the Fusiliers, the loss of their RMO was as bitter as any death.

For Major Geoffrey Hardwick the first sign of the new offensive was that beer prices in the officers' mess went up. Then he was ordered to lead his 59th Field Ambulance to a new location alongside the 19th Division. The field ambulance was one of the mobile aid posts, made up of carts and mule trains. With its own MOs and bearer teams, it could be sent wherever it was needed. Moving up and down the line wherever trouble flared, rather than waiting for it to catch up with them, it collected and treated casualties.[12] The 59th waited for a few days at its new location and then, on 1 July 1916, it was off, the following days and nights blurring into one bloody whole.

Ten days later they were moved again, this time to a location alongside a small railway line that had been built specially for the offensive. Hardwick was told that his casualties were only fourth in line for use of a trolley to get them back to a CCS. The first priority was shells, the next Royal Engineers' supplies, then rations; last, and definitely least, came the wounded. The only entries in Hardwick's diary during the first weeks of the Somme read: 'dead men + +'. He even gave up trying to read and just sat in his dugout when he was off duty, smoking pipe after pipe, his nights filled with the unending thump-thumping of shells landing nearby.

Unlike troops who were moved back and forth from trench to billet, the field ambulances were kept close to the front for as long as possible. The 59th saw service from the very first day of the Somme to the last, 19 November. It moved from Guillemont to Ginchy, Morval and Martinpuich, and then to Thiepval, Le Transloy and the sodden valley of the Ancre.[13] For Hardwick, it was all one and the same, except for a growing danger from abandoned munitions that increasingly cluttered the roads and landscape through which they moved. Even the thousands of empty shell cases half-buried in the mud were a danger, as they could trip up man or horse, breaking a leg or turning over a cart full of supplies and casualties. Then there were the dud bombs and unexploded shells that littered the landscape; there were so many that you stopped noticing them after a while, until the sound of an explosion served as a reminder. Sappers tried to clear areas of munitions, but no one had time to get rid of the miles and miles of tangled barbed wire and cables that sprawled everywhere. Entire days were wasted as orderlies and bearers had to cut paths through the debris, the wire snagging and ripping their clothes and flesh as they worked to make a way for the field ambulance.

By September 1916, Hardwick was beginning to think that the battle would never end and that he would spend the rest of his life here. He became grateful for small mercies, like the dugout they built in the underground oven of an old bakery at the Stuff Redoubt. It was so deep, and the walls so thick, that they sat in complete silence and in a soft darkness lit up by candles throwing shadows on the solid stone walls. Nobody wanted to return to the harsh light and infernal din of the battle. By now the main assault on Thiepval was over, but the fighting continued, providing a steady stream of casualties to be brought to safety. Hardwick had to find the best route for the bearers to bring them out, so he spent a day scouting the forward area to produce a map with directions from the trenches at Zollern to the Stuff Redoubt. It wasn't a particularly long carry, about two hours, but without some kind of map the bearers would get lost in the blasted land-scape of the battlefield. Hardwick kept the instructions simple, providing landmarks that they would all recognise:

Trip from Zollern to Stuff in order:
1. Trench board over a wide trench
2. Then make due N for a smashed up harrow
3. A smashed Bosche lumber cart in a shell hole
4. Then two dead Huns also lying in a shell hole and then 50 yards in front we drop into trench leading to Stuff Road.

In November, when most of the world thought the battle of the Somme was over, Hardwick and the men of the 59th Field Ambulance knew it was not. Each day seemed grimmer and more pointless than the last. They had moved from the safe bakery into a new dugout that was at best only splinterproof. To make matters worse, a heavy rainstorm had washed away some of the walls, revealing the corpses of six Germans in one parapet. By now Hardwick was struggling to support his staff. Several bearers would go sick each day from the strain of holding up for months on end under the stress of battle. Yet despite his sympathy for the men, Hardwick brooked no argument. Sick meant sick, and anything else meant that you worked as normal. If he let one fall out, the whole lot would disappear.

Besides, they were all in it together. They had very little water and had received no supplies of clean, new clothes for weeks. There was no prospect of replacement for tunics ripped by barbed wire, so they had to sew them back together themselves. There seemed to be as many rats in the dugouts as lice on their bodies, and ration deliveries were sporadic and inadequate. They received little news of the progress of the battle, except what they heard from the walking wounded who turned up at the dugout for treatment. Their stories of scores of wounded men, out near the front, which the bearers had no hope of reaching, did little to lift their mood. By the time the offensive officially came to a halt on 19 November, the 59th was barely able to crawl back towards the rear, with its prospect of food, water and a thorough clean.

Perhaps in recognition of their long exposure to the worst of the war, the field ambulance was held back from the front for most of 1917. They were based at a casualty clearing station, and such was their comfort and sense of security that in late spring Hardwick attached a makeshift plough to his horse and created a small vegetable garden. It was a fertile spot, thanks also to the horse, and the neat little rows of green shoots emerging from the manure-rich soil contrasted with the devastated remains of a small town nearby. Hardwick was now able to treat a much wider range of medical ailments than he was used to, including patients in a new influenza ward. He even became a kind of GP to the few locals left behind, helping to deliver a baby and getting paid in cheap local wine.

He was also able to study men with a range of psychiatric conditions brought on by the war, who were kept in a separate tent at the CCS. All over the front RMOs were coming to find this class of patient increasingly interesting. For some of them the treatment was quite simple: when the sound of the guns drew nearer and the patients became increasingly upset, the staff went round the ward putting cotton wool in their ears to muffle the noise and restore calm.[14] Later on that year Hardwick was summoned to testify at the court martial of one of his former patients in the mental ward, who had been arrested for desertion. For nearly an hour the army prosecutor kept Hardwick in the witness box, asking him the most blithering questions he had ever heard on a subject that the army lawyer evidently didn't understand. Then he was dismissed. Hardwick never found out what happened to the man, but feared the worst.[15]

By January 1918 the 59th Field Ambulance was ready to return to the front line. Hardwick thought it a miracle that they had survived with so few losses. As the array of carts and horses moved out towards another offensive in the Somme valley, it still comprised the same men he had around him since the foundation of the 59th in 1915. And there was no one he would rather go forward with. The war awaited them with some fresh twists. It rained throughout January and most of the brand-new trenches were full to the brim with freezing water; anyone who fell in could easily drown. It also meant that the bearers had to forgo safety below ground, instead having to go all the way over the top for stretcher cases.

When the waters receded, a different plague was sent to try them. Rats by the hundred scuttled freely around the trenches, feeding on all the rubbish left behind by the flood. The men loathed them above all else, and one animal in particular: a huge specimen that waddled where it liked and chewed with impunity. Their hearing became sensitised to the smallest of scratching sounds, which indicated that one of the rats was at work on a boot, a carefully saved biscuit or a candle end. Hardwick was determined to do something about this.

In March he was given a two-week pass, long enough to go all the way home to the West Country to see his family. While he was there he bought two ferrets and a large cage.[16] On the train to London, and at his hotel, noses were wrinkled, but Hardwick dusted the cuffs of his uniform and glared back. The ferrets couldn't have made a better start when they got to the 59th: bombing out of their cages, they returned to place the giant rat dead at Hardwick's feet. It was better than getting a medal. From then on, the ferrets boarded in their own dugout in a nearby shell hole and were released daily. They never failed to find their prey – ten or twenty rats a day sometimes, with thirty five being the record. When the division moved as a result of the German spring offensive, the first order of business was to scoop up the ferrets and stow their cage safely among the medical supplies. On Hardwick's birthday they celebrated with red wine, games of poker and organised ratting, with each kill being celebrated with increasingly drunken cheers and songs about the only two creatures who really enjoyed themselves on the Western Front. What would the ferrets do, the men wondered, if the war ever ended? How could they ever go back to a Cornish farm, now that they had hunted for trench rats in France?

By April 1918 the 59th Field Ambulance was back on the old battlefield of the Somme. It looked much the same as it had when they had left at the end of 1916. There were still empty shell casings scattered and half-buried, and tangles of barbed wire as far as the eye could see. And almost the same numbers of wounded men. But this time the field ambulance itself would not escape injury. On 17 April a shell hit its medical post, burying it under tons of wet mud. Sharples, Hardwick's lead bearer, was killed instantly along with two others, and Hardwick dug for hours to free another five men. They had survived together for three years, but now the field ambulance was finally broken apart. Hardwick stayed on until the war ended in November. Then he and his ferrets quietly returned home.

Charles McKerrow had been a GP in Ayr before volunteering for the RAMC in May 1915 and being appointed RMO to the 10th Battalion Northumberland Fusiliers. He went despite his wife Jean's misgivings, but felt he had no choice. Others might have sheltered behind their practice or some ailment, but he knew he would never have been able to live with himself if he had done the same. He didn't quite put it in those terms to Jean. He lied to her instead: he would hardly be in any danger at all, he wrote. Doctors were not allowed to advance with the first line of the regiment. He was expressly forbidden, by the most stringent 'regulations', to put himself in harm's way. He was mostly to hide himself amongst the baggage. And just in case she didn't quite believe him, he wrote to her almost every day, even if it was just one of those pre-printed postcards saying that he was well.

McKerrow's first billet was in a ruined farmhouse in Laventie. It had so many bullet holes in its tin roof that it looked like a pepper pot. His bearer teams and orderlies had come to the farmhouse to meet him and there were moments of nervous tension as they waited to discover what kind of man the new RMO would be. It didn't take them long to work McKerrow out. When they arrived, he was in his shirt sleeves, carrying some carpentry tools and planks. He'd been given the worst kind of little cart, he explained, just a bit of wood with four wheels nailed to the sides. No use to anyone – everything fell off. What was needed was something with sides and a bit of shelving, and a few handholds. It should be able to carry at least three patients and some supplies. He talked and listened to his bearers and orderlies while he worked on his cart and, when he had finished, they saw that he had built just what he had said he would. No need to worry about the new doc.

For his part, McKerrow also liked what he found. There were three men in particular whom he came to rely on. Clark and

Kirtley headed up a team of thirty-two bearers, and Matthew Coulson was the chief orderly, who would look after McKerrow personally. The new RMO gave his weekly lectures to the bearer teams and found them so receptive that by November he had encouraged them to treat slight cases themselves in the nearest trench. As it got colder and wetter, his lectures focused on the problem of trench foot, explaining its causes and the preventative measures. The bearers listened intently and decided to take the message out to the soldiers. Organising themselves into small groups, they put together specialist supply panniers and visited every single one of the Northumberlands' trenches. There they lectured and then saw each case of trench foot, treating it and demonstrating care of the condition to the entire battalion.

McKerrow was extremely proud of them. He was also grateful, for he needed all the spare time he could get, not just for writing to Jean, but because the local people had discovered the doctor billeted in the old farmhouse. All of a sudden he was a GP again, treating pneumonia and toothache, and birthing babies; he was even summoned by the local farmer when three of his cows were injured by a shell exploding in his barn. The locals couldn't pay him, but they did his laundry and replaced the straw bedding that his horse, Tommy, consumed every day.

It wasn't just the locals who helped McKerrow. RAMC supply lines in his area were unreliable, so he turned to a source he knew to be efficient: his wife back in Ayr. She'd already sent him provisions – tinned sardines, haggis and shortbread – and when he asked her to 'join the team', she agreed. Jean soon found him the lice combs and medical scissors that he needed, ordering in bulk. Bearers lost scissors every time they went on a carry, so there were plenty of repeat orders. She also got shirts and socks for those men who couldn't get to a laundry. As the first Christmas approached, she sent vegetables, ham and kippers. This enabled McKerrow to care for his men to the best of his ability, as the RAMC instructed him, but he couldn't have done it without his wife.[17]

The first time McKerrow saw his dugout in the trenches he was amazed at how well dug it was. When he met his men of the Northumberlands he found out why: most of them were miners and, when it came to repairing trenches, digging sanitary pits, wells or RMOs' dugouts, they were second to none. They enjoyed the work because it took them away from the boredom of sentry duty and trench life. On a chilly evening one of them suggested that he put a fireplace in one of the larger medical dugouts. When the doc returned a few days later there was indeed a fireplace dug into the wall, brick-lined and with a chimney to let out the smoke.

Over Christmas and into the New Year the Northumberlands were involved in several attacks. It had rained heavily and they were unable to drain the water out of the trenches and dugouts. Everyone wore waders wherever they were – hard enough to get out of when you were fishing, McKerrow thought, never mind just about to go over the top. If anything was dropped in the mud, it sank, never to be seen again; McKerrow lost a pair of slippers that way. He even had to raise up his bed on wooden planks to lift it away from the water.

Conditions were taking their toll. His entire world seemed to consist of the reeking aid post and the freezing, sodden battle front; there were days when McKerrow could hardly remember anything else. Yet Jean's parcels always contained something personal from her and the family – a photograph, a hand-warmer, a copy of the *Ayrshire Post* – which cheered him up. In return he asked her if she wanted any polished-brass shrapnel noses to use as vases in their living room.

And sometimes there was even good news at the front. One day word came from a nearby CCS that a man whose life McKerrow and the bearer teams had worked particularly hard to save had indeed survived. McKerrow made sure to tell each member of the bearer team personally. That night he walked out into the open and looked up at the stars. It was a clear night, and to his surprise he found that he could quite easily see Venus and Jupiter just setting, and Mars and Saturn rising. A busy night, astronomically. Back in his dugout he wrote down his

observations. From then on, with stellar charts sent by Jean, he became one of many men and women at the front who looked up towards the heavens and found comfort in the eternal passage of the stars.

McKerrow's reputation as a fine RMO soon began to spread. Men from other battalions sought him out, if their own doctor wasn't available – and sometimes even if he was, turning up to his sick parades trying to blend in. He made a point of going round the lines every single day, and several times if there were new arrivals to the battalion, realising that newcomers became agitated if they thought the doctor hadn't noticed them. He found that he had come to prefer trenches to billets, and wrote home to Jean that when he came back to Ayr he would probably always walk in the gutter. It wasn't the only thing that surprised him. Sometimes he almost forgot about the war. Once, treating the wounded under fire for hours on end, he simply stopped noticing the sound of the guns and worked as calmly as if he were in his examination rooms at home.

In May 1916, McKerrow was informed of the forthcoming offensive. He was ordered to reduce his personal belongings to a minimum and was moved to a new aid post and billet near Amiens. He was aware of the seriousness of the situation and, in a letter accompanying a parcel of his belongings he assured his wife that during the next three months he would be cautious to excess.[18] His battalion didn't join the Somme offensive until the end of the first week. By then it had heard what had happened to three other Northumberland battalions. Attacking La Boisselle on the first day of the battle, they had lost 2,440 men and seventy officers within hours.[19] When their own battalion finally went forward, McKerrow set up an aid post as close to the new front as possible. He followed the troops as they moved forward, at one point taking over a German aid post, complete with casualties and a medical orderly, who insisted on helping him.

McKerrow worked for three straight days, treating 1,000 casualties without stopping. They came in and went out again, and

piles of bloodied bandages were trampled down into the mud, layer on layer. Watching over him was his orderly, Matt Coulson, who brought him continual supplies of coffee and soup, chasing after him round the aid post until McKerrow took the mug and drank whatever he was given. Coulson also brought fresh socks for the doctor, and made him sit down in a corner while he changed them and rubbed his feet and legs. But he couldn't keep the RMO off his feet for long. Only on 10 July did McKerrow retire to the rear for a brief rest. In his first letter home to Jean his pride in his team, three of whom would later receive medals, took precedence over his own experience:

> No one could have possibly equalled my stretcher bearers . . . As one hard-bitten chap said to me, 'they are doing Christ's work'. It really is very fine to see these chaps passing through storms of shell to help their comrades. I am very proud of them and hope they will get some rewards apart from the normal ones of their conscience.

In the third week of July the pace of battle slowed. Pushing further forward into enemy territory, the Northumberlands stumbled upon an artillery officer's dugout, which they duly presented to their RMO to serve as an aid post. McKerrow had a good look through the things that the German officer had left behind, before lighting a fire and making coffee for Coulson and some of the bearers; he imagined how annoying it must be for the previous occupant to see smoke puffing up into the sky from his old dugout. McKerrow had spent a year in Vienna as part of his medical training and spoke fluent German, so when he found a cache of letters he translated them for Jean. She could see what a German officer – a man not so different from him – might write home.

At the end of July he was summoned to the rear to take part in the court martial of one of the casualties he had treated during the first three days, who had been accused of inflicting the wound on himself. Taking the witness stand on behalf of the soldier, McKerrow remembered quite clearly that there had been no

powder burns on either the man's skin or on any of the clothes that he had been wearing. In which case, he stated, the shot must have been fired from some distance away. His cool scientific testimony ensured that the man was acquitted.

He returned to the front to find that he had lost his comfortable German dugout in an enemy counterattack, and for the next two weeks the Northumberlands moved back and forth. McKerrow moved from aid post to aid post, and onto the field of battle itself. Once again, the days blurred into each other. He realised that somehow death had become unimportant to him. It wasn't callousness, just too much knowledge. He had other problems to solve. When one morning during battle there was no time to dig a new aid post, he went round the battalion and borrowed all the men's greatcoats. Then he found a deep shell hole and constructed a roof with the coats held up by rifles. The Northumberlands looked on in amazement, and McKerrow's reputation for fearlessness and ingenuity grew even more.

By mid-August he was the only RMO left in the entire brigade and his bearer teams were badly depleted. There was barely enough time to train up their replacements, but somehow Kirtley and Clark managed to pull them into shape. McKerrow received a letter from Jean with the news that an uncle of his had been wounded by shotgun fire on a grouse moor. For the first time in months he got angry: as if there weren't enough places in the world to get shot. One attack by the Northumberlands had cost the lives of two-thirds of the men taking part. That night he went out with the bearer teams to bring in the wounded and lost a bearer to a sniper. McKerrow knew the danger he put himself in, but his duty was not only to the wounded, but also to the unharmed soldiers in the battalion. They attacked with far greater confidence if they knew that he and his bearer teams would come to find and treat them.

October was a low point for McKerrow. Tommy, the scruffy horse that had carried him and pulled his cart for more than a year, attacked a groom and had to be destroyed. The stress of battle had got to the animal, as it had to the humans around him. Everywhere McKerrow looked there was loss. By now his entire bearer teams consisted of replacements, with only Clark and Kirtley surviving. They had been moved again, into an area where there was almost constant fighting. One of the new intake was shot in the stomach by a sniper almost as soon as he arrived. For the first time McKerrow began to wonder if he had now done his duty and felt it might be time to move to a safer position in the rear. He had a friend who ran a field hospital and made an informal enquiry to him about a transfer.

When the battalion was moved again to a quiet part of the front and the offensive finally ended, McKerrow had time to work on another project that he had taken on. Trench fever was a type of flu that brought down men by the hundreds for days at a time, without any discernible infectious agent. Always more interested in the defeat of the microbe than in that of the human enemy, McKerrow began to investigate the root causes and conditions of the disease. To Jean fell the task of going through all the diaries he had kept since his arrival in France and had sent back to her in Ayr, in which he had recorded the weather and general medical statistics from his brigade. Whilst Jean processed the data, Kirtley made a significant personal contribution to the research by going down with trench fever himself. He was installed on a stretcher in McKerrow's dugout, so that he and the doc could study every aspect of his illness. McKerrow was the first RMO in France to research the condition and wrote up his research into a paper, 'Pyrexias of Doubtful Origin in an Infantry Battalion on Active Service'. When he read it at an RAMC conference to great acclaim, he was asked to prepare it for publication.[20]

This response to his work gave him new heart, and for the first time since the beginning of the Somme offensive his letters home became more positive. He even started imagining life after the war, planning a long family trip to India. He formalised his request to transfer to a field hospital and applied for some leave – he hadn't been home since April. It was the longest separation from

Jean since they were married and he was especially looking forward to seeing his son; he even contemplated diagnosing the boy with a mysterious ailment so that he could extend his time at home for a few more days.

On 20 December, McKerrow and Clark left the aid post for their daily tour of the line. They never got to their men. At ten o'clock an enemy shell exploded close to them and both medics were hit. Horrified Northumberlands gathered around them and a bearer party, including Matt Coulson, arrived immediately. The two men were taken by stretcher to their own aid post and from there by ambulance to the nearest casualty clearing station four miles away. Their supply of morphine was good and there were few bumps in the road, yet both men had ruptures to all the major abdominal arteries and their conditions were inoperable. Clark died soon after arriving at the CCS, with Matt Coulson at his side. McKerrow was nursed by a fellow Scot, Sister Constance Druce, and he impressed her with his great calm and his refusal to fear the inevitable. He died at nine o'clock that evening.

The next day the bodies of McKerrow and Clark were wrapped in blankets and buried in the little cemetery in Poperinghe. For the men of the 10th Battalion it was the worst loss they had experienced and they decided to honour their RMO by building a cross for him and erecting it over his grave. Many of them wrote to Jean with their condolences, but Coulson couldn't bear setting pen to paper. Instead his wife wrote to McKerrow's widow, woman to woman, explaining that her husband was overcome with grief and couldn't yet bring himself to talk about the loss.

As McKerrow would have wished it, Jean oversaw the publication of his article on trench fever in the 1918 volume of the *Journal of the Royal Army Medical Corps*. Coulson became the orderly-servant to the battlion's new RMO, who would later record that, for the remainder of the war, Coulson talked of little else but Doc McKerrow.

4

Surgeons

Henry Souttar, Norman Pritchard, John Hayward

We hope that our humble attempts may at least show that five miles behind the trenches there is room for the highest surgical skill that England can produce.

Henry Souttar, January 1915[1]

When war broke out, Henry Souttar immediately volunteered his services.[2] He had much to offer. He was a fine, experienced surgeon at a large, modern London teaching hospital. He had grown up in the new age of surgery, with antiseptics and white-tiled operating rooms, well lit and fully staffed, in hospitals containing all the necessary support facilities. Moreover, he had served in South Africa, so he knew what modern war looked like. A man of his quality was noticed immediately, and Souttar was posted to Antwerp to run a large hospital, fully equipped and staffed by the Red Cross, for casualties from the Belgian Army. It had been particularly satisfying to watch his staff unpack one of the latest innovations, an instrument steriliser, and Souttar followed them to the operating theatre to watch it being set it up. It seemed to sum up all his hopes and expectations for the new hospital – the No. 1 Belgian Field.

But almost as soon as Souttar had settled in, the German Army headed towards Antwerp. The front was supposed to be too far away to worry about, but soon it arrived almost at their doorstep. First his wards filled beyond capacity, then a shell landed in the garden of the hospital. Souttar was ordered to evacuate. One of the London double-decker buses, converted for service at the front, was sent to collect the medical staff and their patients to join the trek west. They were about to set off when an orderly noticed that Souttar wasn't on board. He was spotted dragging the steriliser down the front steps, determined to save it, but when another shell hit the main building he finally gave up and ran for his life. The steriliser, symbol of his hopes and optimism, was left behind in the driveway, with dust and debris starting to settle on its glass surfaces.

The Germans chased Souttar out of Antwerp and into the last corner of unoccupied Belgium, defended by a remnant Belgian Army. He could only watch as casualty numbers increased. But then the Red Cross told him that they had found a site for a new hospital, in Furnes on the banks of the River Yser. It was relatively safe and the building had once been a theological college, with sturdy walls and plenty of dormitory rooms. It wouldn't be like Antwerp, but they would get all the supplies to him that they could. The No. 1 Belgian Field was reborn.

When Souttar and his staff of nurses, orderlies and ambulance drivers arrived in Furnes, their spirits sank. The old college was filthy. Everything was covered in dust and the windows were black with soot. Yes, the dormitories could be made up into wards, but they found only twelve beds. The building's long, narrow corridors and unlit stairways were difficult to navigate. Souttar searched the entire building to find a room that would be suitable for an operating theatre. The one he eventually picked would need painting and furnishing from the bits and pieces littered about the place, but for the time being a good clean would have to do. But there wasn't any great hurry. Only one box of supplies had so far arrived; they couldn't do much for anyone at this stage, so they might as well wait and get on with the scrubbing down.

When the nurses opened the windows to let in light and air, they could hear the guns in the distance. It was an ominous sign. No hospital could function properly so close to the front. Then they heard the sound of lorry engines. Hurrying into the courtyard, they thought their supplies had finally arrived. Instead ten ambulances pulled up, one after another, parking next to the still-unpacked staff suitcases. Souttar rushed out and found each vehicle full of badly wounded men. They weren't ready, he told the drivers – they had no equipment. But even as he spoke the words he realised that if no one treated these men, they would die. They were a hospital, and now they had patients. The work would begin at once.

Orderlies and drivers began to unload the stretchers and line them up in the courtyard. Then another engine was heard coming down the road. This time it was one of their lorries and it brought some of their supplies: dressings, drugs and anaesthetic equipment. Souttar mustered a surgical team and sent them to the new operating theatre. He chose the first patient from the men lined up on stretchers, put on his gown and followed him as he was carried into surgery. His staff had lined up neatly on a tray all the equipment they could find. In addition to the drugs and dressings, he had two scalpels, six artery forceps, two dissecting forceps and a finger saw. It was almost laughable, but it would have to do. Then, with the stretcher laid across a table, he set to work on his first patient.

That evening Souttar stood at the door of his new postoperative ward and looked at the results of the day's work. Men slept on the few beds and on palliasses – mattresses made of ticking or sheeting sewn around fresh straw – with blankets and pillows scrounged from somewhere or belonging to the nurses. A few gas lamps gave off a soft, low light and the sturdy wooden window frames were keeping the sound of the war away. Souttar listened for a while to the sounds of men sleeping, breathing, murmuring to themselves. It was hard to believe that these were the same men who had lain on filthy stretchers in the courtyard earlier, with savage abdominal injuries and dreadful bleeding, their bodies full of shrapnel and covered in half the mud of Belgium. Their lives had been reclaimed. From the first incision, the day had been a blur, but he tried to remember what he had done. It was important to turn chaos into reason.

One by one they had been brought to him, and one by one he had operated in dim light and with the most basic equipment. He repaired ruptured veins and arteries and saved lives with just a few stitches. He cleared away debris blown deep into ragged wounds. He stitched up torn faces and hands. He set broken bones and joints. He excised and debrided infected flesh so that wounds could heal cleanly. He tackled severe abdominal injuries, sometimes in utter disbelief that he was able to work like this outside a modern hospital.

After very little sleep, Souttar returned to theatre in the morning. He worked for two more days, until no more ambulances came round the corner and no more men lay on stretchers in the courtyard. Not all of them could be saved, and every death was crushing. But Souttar tried to reassure his staff: had they not opened the hospital – had they not tried – every single man now in their care would have died on the road to the coast. So despite the lack of equipment, of mattresses, of light, and despite the bodies stacked in a cool outhouse to the rear of the hospital awaiting the sanitary squads, No. 1 Belgian Field had been a success.[3] They had saved the lives of so many men, some within an hour of their wounding. No base hospital ever saw the kind of casualty they did. What they were doing was unprecedented.

By the end of January 1915 Souttar and his staff had treated more than 1,000 patients.[4] While the operating theatre ran late into the night, the nurses and orderlies gradually improved the rest of the hospital. More beds and mattresses were procured. The kitchen was equipped, staff dormitories were allocated. An electrical supply was connected to the operating theatre and some of the wards. Nobody tripped on the stairs any more, after a wealthy nurse bought boxes of lamps and oil in town and hung them on every dark stairwell and down all the corridors.

But however hard they tried, there was simply no comparison with the hospital they had abandoned in Antwerp. They had to endure the terrible smell of the incinerator burning bloody dressings and linen. And the sight of a row of corpses waiting to be moved. All they could do was learn to look the other way when they passed through the courtyard. They tried not to be crushed by the sheer number of ambulances, each arriving with their pitiful shelves laden with wounded men, but for some it was too much. One volunteer could no longer cope with unloading and was put on ambulance cleaning duty. But even the sight of an empty vehicle, with its puddles of congealing blood and saturated dressings clumped on the floor, was too much for her, and Souttar had to send her home.[5] And all the time, lorries rumbled past on the road outside with fresh fodder for the ever-pounding guns.

Yet they did at last feel safe. The Belgian king had ordered the sluice gates to be opened on the River Yser and the plain on its far bank had been flooded; there could be no enemy advance through miles of yard-deep swamp. So they had their own moat – an odd one, to be sure: brackish, oil-slicked and with all manner of floating debris slowly drifting past.[6] They were the most forward hospital in their part of the line, and everyone at the front knew it. During battles, the hospital was permanently at full capacity, with 350 patients and many more waiting on stretchers for beds. Furnes had a large railway station, so as soon as they were strong enough, patients were put on ambulance trains to Calais.

Just as Souttar learned in the operating theatre (now painted white and with the proper complement of trollies and instruments), so his nurses learned in the wards. Their lessons were every bit as fundamental. In Antwerp their patients had been strong enough to survive long ambulance journeys, none of them being at risk from dehydration, shock or bleeding to death. Yet those arriving in Furnes were often dying of those very conditions, never mind the wounds themselves. It was up to the nurses to treat them before they were ready for surgery. They had all been trained in resuscitation techniques, but had rarely got a chance to practise them. Now they did.

Within weeks of their arrival in Furnes, Souttar's nurses had developed a resuscitation protocol that, as far as the surgical team was concerned, brought the dead back to life. The worst of the mud was cleaned off the patient before he was laid down on a mattress and hot-water bottles placed all around him to warm him up. Then he was given warm saline intravenously and, once he could raise his head, spoonfuls of hot coffee, fortified with brandy. Next came morphine in quarter-grain doses until his pain was gone. The nurses watched closely, modifying their treatment if necessary, until the drawn, grey face of the patient turned pink, his breathing deepened and slowed, and a muddy hand clutched theirs in wordless thanks.[7] Souttar never failed to marvel at what his nurses were doing. It was the real work of the hospital.

Souttar felt he had been able to tackle almost everything thrown at him at No. 1 Belgian Field. Nothing surprised him much any more, although he could still amaze his own nurses. There was the intact time-fuse lodged under a shoulder blade, or the length of watch chain that he pulled out of a leg wound, link by link, like a sideshow magician.[8] And now that he had a team he could really rely on, he started to think about what else the hospital might need. His plans received a boost from their excellent patron, the Belgian queen.[9] When Queen Elizabeth came to visit she always arrived with lorryloads of supplies requested by Souttar. And it was the queen who finally got the last of the straw palliasses replaced with real beds and ensured that their store cupboards were full of linen, pillows and blankets. And, once word of the royal patronage got out in Furnes, the locals rallied round to help. Supplies of food became more regular, and five nuns arrived from the nearby convent to help in the kitchen and laundry.

The kitchen was becoming the heart of the entire place, mostly due to a Belgian soldier called Maurice. Souttar had treated Maurice for a serious throat wound and then 'prescribed' time in the kitchen, with its warm, damp atmosphere, to continue the healing process. Soon Maurice made himself useful at the stove, cooking over the huge pots and producing a delicious thick and yeasty stew, quite unlike the plain, watery fare produced by the nuns. What Maurice could do with bully beef and stock bones was almost as miraculous as what the nurses did with coffee and brandy. It turned out that before he was conscripted, Maurice had been a sous-chef at the Hôtel Métropole in Brussels, so Souttar exercised his power to retain a patient and turned the kitchen over to him. Soon the nurses took all their breaks there, gathering and laughing round the warm ovens, with the sound of Maurice's tin-whistle laughter at the heart of it all.

During the warm summer of 1915 the nurses pitched tents in the grounds around the hospital and slept outside. One day they had a special visitor. When a stocky little van pulled up in the courtyard, it turned out to be the mobile radiology laboratory of Professor Marie Curie.[10] As an amateur physics buff, Souttar was familiar with her work and explained to his staff that the professor believed that the lack of X-ray facilities at the front was killing men who might otherwise be saved. She had therefore set up a fleet of mobile radiology labs, in converted Renault vans that she paid for herself. She had trained a corps of radiographers and they were installing the labs at all the most forward medical facilities. Now the great lady herself had come to the No. 1 Belgian Field.

After introductions and a short demonstration of the van, it was decided that the best place for the new lab would be in a dressing room next to the operating theatre in the old stable block. Under the curious eyes of the nurses and orderlies, Curie hooked up the generator and the cables and built up the radiology unit, piece by piece. She carefully stacked boxes of replacement films and explained how the pens should not be used elsewhere, as they had special ink in them so that they could be used to write on the shiny surface of the film. Finally she was finished. Where would she sleep? Souttar hadn't anticipated that the great lady would be staying. Would she mind sharing a tent in the garden?[11]

The next day Curie escorted her first patient to the lab and took his X-rays while Souttar and the theatre staff watched and listened. When the patient was moved to the operating room, they were able to extract all the shrapnel fragments peppering his body in one go. Previously surgeons had to wait and observe as these éclats slowly made themselves known through pain and infection, and the patient had to endure multiple surgery to get them all out.[12] Souttar was delighted that Curie stayed on at the hospital for several more weeks. To have her at his side as he worked, conferring and discussing, was a blessing. She probably stayed longer than she had planned, for not every surgeon appreciated her work in the same way. Some accepted the gift of the lab and waved her on, but there was no question of letting an unqualified woman – even one with a Nobel Prize – anywhere near the theatre. Souttar felt very differently, and the professor repaid his faith every day. Curie was not just an expert in radiology: she was a competent engineer and performed all sorts of jobs to do with wiring or mechanics around the hospital. When, during her stay, a high-ranking Belgian general was brought in, she rigged up a telephone line to his bedside so that he could speak to the king and the Army Council.

In the spring of 1916 Souttar was recalled home as consultant surgeon to the Southern Command, based at Netley. It was a significant promotion and a worthy recognition of his achievements. He hadn't been the only surgeon to find himself so close to the front line, but he had been one of the first to demonstrate his abilities and pass on the lessons he had learned. He would now be at the very heart of the planning for the forthcoming offensive.

After he left most of his staff moved on to other hospitals or returned to Britain. The Belgian Army took over the running of the hospital and the senior positions were filled by their surgeons. In time for the summer offensive, staff numbers were considerably increased. And as these new arrivals jumped down from their lorries and found their way to the staff dormitory, they would have assumed that the hospital had always been there, just behind the guns, to treat the wounded close to where they fell. A place where they could stop death in its tracks.[13]

Norman Pritchard had been a police surgeon in London before the war, so he felt that there wasn't much that would shock him when he got to the front. It was the early summer of 1915 and he was pleased with his posting to one of the all-new casualty clearing stations – No. 3 – with its purpose-built operating theatres and long tented wards. He could see for himself how quickly the lessons from the war's first few months had been learned. It was as if as much of a London hospital as possible had been picked up and moved close to the front.

For No. 3 the front was Ypres, and the war could never keep away from Ypres for very long. The second battle of that name had broken out just before Pritchard arrived. He was rarely out of his surgical scrubs for the first two weeks. In his tent, late at night, he tried to write up his diary, to make sense of it all. On the third night, when he read it back to himself, he found that he had only written of the many dozens of amputations he had undertaken in the last few days. Field ambulances and RMOs had been ordered not to amputate except in extreme cases, so the decisions to sever limbs were almost all being made at the CCSs by surgeons like Pritchard.[14] Orderlies had been gathering up limbs like logs for the fire and taking them away. He had no idea what they did with them at No. 3. Was there a pit for burying human debris, or did they use an incinerator? Pritchard hadn't yet come to grips with the layout of the place: the only path he travelled was that between the operating tent and his billet. He had assumed, from civilian practice, that amputations were a thing of the past, but here he was, gore-stained and exhausted, serving on an assembly line of sawing and hacking. He heard that surgical instruments wore out so quickly at the front that cutlers' shops had been set up on a permanent basis nearby to sharpen them.[15] It didn't surprise him. It was too much to think about it all, so he worked on, day after day, until the second battle of Ypres ended a few weeks later on.

If Pritchard thought there would be time to rest once the German offensive had failed, he was mistaken. British troops had rounded up all the wounded Germans left behind on the battlefield and now they were bringing them to No. 3. When Pritchard first set eyes on them, in their special ward, he almost turned round and walked out again. The POWs were in a dreadful state. Most had been in hiding for days, lying in abandoned trenches and shell holes, hoping that their side would retake the ground. They were fetid with infections and starved, many of them on the brink of death. It was difficult to know where to start. Pritchard had no German, and so a kind, firm tone would have to do.

He first tried to remove the remains of their uniforms, so that the cleaning and treatment of their wounds could begin. Gradually his patients began to relax, most too overwhelmed by exhaustion to resist any further. They were fed a little at a time and given water; then the orderlies started to wash away the mud and blood from their bodies. CCS staff who were German speakers dropped in to help out. There were small exchanges in German and English and nervous, desperate smiles. But by the end of the first day the prisoners were clean, bandaged and in bed, and the tent began to smell like any other ward. Pritchard watched as one of his orderlies carried away a mound of rags and soiled dressings for incineration. Then he nodded to the guard posted outside and returned to his own tent.

The next day was much more normal. He went round each POW bed, wrote up tickets and instructed the orderlies on who would be needing operations. By now his patients had accepted that they were in a hospital and no one resisted as they were taken away for anaesthetics and surgery. During his round that evening Pritchard looked around him and realised he had quite forgotten that it was a POW ward. It was a satisfying thought and he stayed for a while longer, pleased to see men coming back to life.

But as suddenly as they had arrived, a fleet of lorries came to take his patients away. There were new camps, he learned, well to the rear, with plenty of hospital space for those still in need of care. As Pritchard watched the lorries drive away, he realised that he finally had time to explore No. 3 in its entirety. Both the receiving and the operating tents were empty; the only place still busy was the sick ward, with beds full of men with hacking coughs, fevers and worse. Its patients had conditions that Pritchard had previously treated only in children, such as measles and mumps – mostly the result of too many men living too closely together.

Pritchard went back to the sick ward over the next few days and realised how much he missed being busy. If there were no wounded, then the sick would have to do. No one really wanted to work on the sick ward, but from the outset Pritchard found it interesting. He treated measles, meningitis, diphtheria, scabies and all manner of enteric conditions, and as a result became something of a sick-ward specialist in his sector, receiving cases transferred from other CCSs. He worked all through the cold winter of 1915 and on into the spring, receiving some of the very first influenza cases seen at the front. He certainly did not miss those piles of limbs being carried off by the orderlies.

But it was not to last. In May 1916 orders came through that they should prepare themselves for a big push in the summer. No. 3 was moved to a new, expanded site in the middle of hundreds of acres of cornfields near Puchevillers, where it became CCS No. 44. Pritchard wondered how they would get the wounded to them, as the roads seemed hardly adequate. But then he watched as a temporary railway was laid through the corn up to a small railhead: there would be special trains for the wounded and then a short carry up to the CCS. The preparations picked up speed; a pile of stretchers was stacked at the railhead; the sick ward was emptied and there was to be no more leave. A blood-donation tent was set up, although finding donors wasn't easy: healthy men were superstitious about going into the CCS and nervous about giving blood. Only when they were given a pint of stout in exchange for their donation did the blood banks begin to fill.[16]

The first ambulance train arrived on 19 June and, while it wasn't full, the nursing staff were soon busy enough with men injured during the preparation of the battlefield. Then, on 1 July, the battle began. Pritchard took up his station in the operating theatre and

watched as it filled within hours. During the first three days of
the offensive 4,500 wounded men were sent to No. 44. This was
well beyond its capacity, and within twenty-four hours the system
began to fail.

No. 44 did not have an infinite number of beds in its wards,
nor an infinite number of orderlies and bearers. All of them were
needed at the CCS that night, carrying between wards and
theatre, assisting the surgeons and medics, digging graves.
Pritchard knew something had gone badly wrong when, sometime during the first night, the operating tent emptied and no
more men were brought in. He went down to the railhead to
find out what was going on. By now it was midnight, but the
sky was clear and starlit with a bright new moon. The sight was
worse than it had been when the German POWs had arrived. It
had been impossible to communicate that No. 44 was full beyond
capacity, so train after train had pulled up and dumped its load
of wounded around the railhead and in the surrounding fields.
There was no one to meet them, no one to tend them, no one
to carry them away. Pritchard started to count how many were
abandoned there, but gave up when he reached ninety-four.
Wounded and dying men were lying in rows everywhere in the
cornfield. Yet there was an eerie silence. All he could hear was
the wind rustling through the unharvested crop. He walked back
to the operating tent, hoping that somehow some of them would
find their way to him there.

For three more days bearers and orderlies flew between the
wards and the field, but they were only able to make a small
impression on the mass of men lying at the railhead. Then, on
the fourth day, things improved when a battalion of Royal Engineers
arrived to help. It was their first assignment during the offensive
and they were eager to make a difference. They helped the bearers
to empty the cornfield and get the wounded into the receiving
tents and the dead to the cemetery. They also put up a temporary
dressing station right by the railhead, so that medics could begin
treating the men as soon as the next train arrived. No. 44 now had

a system that was fully staffed and working – inasmuch as anything worked during the first week of the Somme.

With no orders to move on, the Engineers made themselves useful. It was easy to see that, despite all the preparations, No. 44 just wasn't big enough for the loads it was being sent. So the Engineers put up rows of new huts, including a new dressing area, and installed electric lights. Every extra bed space they made was taken up almost immediately. During the second week of the offensive Pritchard and the other surgeons worked flat out in the operating tents. The only thing that stopped them was the heavy rain that flooded the floor, so they waited for the water to drain before continuing their work.

The surgeons worked in teams, switching between operating and providing anaesthetics for each other. But if Pritchard thought doing anaesthetics would offer even a little respite, he was wrong. Keeping badly wounded men unconscious was extremely difficult, even for an experienced anaesthetist. If the patient hadn't been given enough chloroform, he could start to come out of the induced coma, not far enough to wake up completely, but far enough to relive his wounding – shouting, crying, with his hands scrabbling in the air to beat away the bullets and the shrapnel hitting him in his dreams. Surgeons dreaded such moments, when the terror of the battlefield found its way into their operating theatre.[17]

On 13 July, No. 44 managed to clear 230 patients at the railhead, their biggest load so far. But another train was waiting a little further down the line, with hundreds more. In the wards, the nurses and orderlies struggled to cope. As soon as one man died, another would take his place in his unchanged bed or on his stretcher. And as the dead filled up the little cemetery built just out of sight in the cornfield, the Engineers had to extend it. On 6 August Pritchard noted that he was again spending an entire afternoon doing amputations. Nothing had changed since the second battle of Ypres. When it was over – if it ever would be – he would find another way to save lives that didn't trap him in an operating tent.

Gradually the load lightened and the Engineers moved on. At the end of September the ambulance trains stopped arriving altogether, and their casualties were brought to them in ambulances and trucks, a few at a time. Pritchard stayed on until December, when he accepted a new posting in Italy. The CCS there had a large sick ward and needed his expertise with the growing number of influenza cases. Pritchard liked his new post. He didn't know when the war might end, but if he never heard another amputation saw grate its way through bone, or had to avert his eyes from a pile of limbs awaiting disposal, that would be enough.

John Hayward was close to retirement when war broke out and worried that he would be deemed too old to see action at the front. He was right to worry. Until the summer of 1918 he served with diligence and commitment in a range of hospitals treating the wounded in Britain, including the Army Hospital at Netley where Henry Souttar had arrived after his promotion from No. 1 Belgian Field. By 1918 the CCS system in France had been refined into an extraordinary medical machine. During battle its doctors and surgeons did work of unprecedented complexity and effectiveness. Every medic in the country wanted to be part of it, and Hayward too longed to be blooded at the Western Front – to fight for a soldier's life with the sound of the guns all around, and to win him back from certain death. When his orders finally came through, it was everything he had hoped for: a CCS posting, close to the action at Amiens, where Allied troops were retaking the territory gained by the Germans during the spring offensive.

As Hayward settled into his new surroundings, he watched thousands of soldiers march past the CCS. They would soon be pushing forward towards the enemy, towards Germany. At long last he felt part of the war. Yet the feeling turned sour when he reported for duty. They would have no casualties for two days, he was told. Time for him to settle in, get to know where everything was in the huge complex and get some rest. As he walked round the CCS he introduced himself to the fellow professionals

who would be his colleagues. All of them had been at the front
for at least two years. They were considerably younger than him,
hardened and alert, and seemed to need very little sleep. Then
there was the obvious lack of military discipline: the codes of
conduct that had structured his work at hospitals in Britain were
nowhere to be found. Everything was different, and Hayward
began to fear that he had made a huge mistake – that he should
have stayed in Britain like the other surgeons of his age.

On his first night of duty Hayward was woken up at 1 a.m.,
when the first ambulances appeared in the distance, and told to
take up station as senior MO in the reception tent. The lights
were dim and Hayward sent an orderly for more gas lamps, but
there was no time: a bearer appeared at the tent doorway, with
a man's arm slung over his shoulder. As soon as the wounded
man was set down, another bearer immediately appeared, then
another, and much too quickly the tent filled up with men, some
on stretchers, some slumped in chairs, others lying on the ground.
Finally, as he had wished for, here were casualties straight from
the battlefield.

Hayward was an experienced surgeon, but he had never seen
such frightful wounds. Under the dried blood, filth and sweat
were stumps where limbs had been blown off, smashed faces and
dreadfully contorted bones. Worse sometimes were those with
only a small visible wound, a nick in the stomach where the bullet
had done its work, discreet and deadly. All his patients' faces were
white from too much fear and too little blood. Yet it struck
Hayward how quiet it was inside the tent. There was no groaning.
Instead he just heard breathing, gasping and the occasional rasp
of a match lighting a cigarette. Many of the men had simply fallen
asleep.

Hayward could have foundered there and then, had it not been
for an experienced orderly who assisted him with whispered directions. First he was to sort the patients: those who could stand or
sit, and whose wounds just needed cleaning and dressing, were
moved to one side so that the orderlies could work on them.

Then Hayward was to go through the stretcher cases: those who had to be operated on went to the pre-op tents; those too weak to go into theatre, but with a good chance of surviving, were sent to the resus tent to be warmed up and given saline and blood transfusions by the nurses. No need to worry about them for the moment. Those for whom there was no hope were quietly moved to one side and taken to the moribund ward. The dead went to their own tent for sorting.

At 7 a.m. Hayward's reception tent was finally empty. For a very short while he allowed himself to feel relief that it was over. But there was to be no rest. At 10 a.m. he was due to begin surgery on the very men he had sent to the operating tent, now that they had been cleaned up, shaved and anaesthetised. He dreaded what was waiting for him, as one of only three surgeons to operate on almost a hundred patients. The orderly sensed what he was thinking and tried to reassure him. They had sent for reinforcements from nearby CCSs, he told Hayward, and surgeons and theatre teams were on their way. And there was time for him to have a wash and get some breakfast.

At 10 a.m. he stepped into the operating tent. There were men laid out on every table. He had never seen so many, and their wounds looked even worse now they were cleaned up. Working alongside his colleagues he removed septic tissue and shrapnel fragments, set bones and repaired veins, muscle and skin. He did all Souttar had done on that first day at Furnes, but even though he had more equipment and drugs, it felt every bit as overwhelming. It was unbearably hot in the tent and it was full of noise and bustle. Everything crowded in on him. He tried not to look over his shoulder so he wouldn't see how many men were still waiting for him. He noticed how slow he was, so much slower than his colleagues. While they were clearing patients off their tables within an hour, he was taking two or three hours per man. It was the worst luck of all, he thought, for a man to end up on his table, rather than another surgeon's. He held their lives in his hands and his hands were shaking from the horror. He tried to gather himself by concentrating on every single step of the surgery he was performing but he only just held himself together.

At 7 p.m. the next day, thirty-six hours after he had gone on duty, Hayward finally finished work in theatre. As he ate his dinner and stumbled to his tent, all he could think was that he must return to England to spare both patients and colleagues his incompetence. Then he fell asleep. He slept so deeply he didn't even dream of the horrors of the day, and when he woke up it was with a new resolve. No day could be as bad as the first. He was going to stay and he was going to learn. There were a few cases left over for him and he got through them without any problems. He began to feel a little more as if he might belong here.

That evening he went for a walk in a nearby forest. Walking amongst the trees he resolved that, whatever happened, he would stay in France. That he would pull himself together and that, no matter what, he would never again panic. As he emerged from the forest into the evening sunlight he saw a column of soldiers marching towards the camp. There was something not quite right about them, he thought. They marched too slowly, in double file, and they were covered in some kind of white dust. As they grew closer he could see that they were all holding onto the shoulder of the man in front of them. His orderly ran over. Hayward was wanted in the reception tent – all hands on deck. The column comprised 200 Australian soldiers and they had all been gassed, the orderly told him. They were all blinded and choking from the fluid in their lungs. Hayward ran to the tent to meet them. All through the night he and the others worked to clean their eyes and wash the dust away. At dawn an orderly led the queue of bandaged men, still shivering from shock and fear of blindness, to the wards to sleep. Hayward went to his own camp bed. He had not panicked. And tomorrow, he resolved, he wouldn't panic either.

Weeks passed and gradually he was becoming as battle-hardened as his colleagues. No one called across to him in theatre any more to tell him what to do. His orderly stopped whispering advice, and the nurses began to seek him out if they had a difficult case to deal with. Then, in the early autumn of 1918, the CCS moved to an abandoned asylum, in support of a new offensive. The place was cramped, dirty and unprepared to receive a fully functioning CCS. They were still waiting for supplies and extra staff when the barrage started up and the first ambulances pulled up in the main courtyard. There were 200 men in the first wave of casualties and another 200 in the second. So packed was the place with stretchers that one orderly spent all his time just making sure a narrow passage was kept in between them, so that the doctors and nurses could pass.

Nine surgeons worked non-stop in the operating theatre, and it seemed to Hayward that their work made little difference. They often went down together to the pre-op room to select the next patients to operate on. Again, Hayward felt each selection like a knife slicing through him. He had been given the power over life and death, by choosing who would be going into surgery. But, like his colleagues, he worked on with desperate determination. And all the while he could hear more ambulances arriving. During a break in surgery he heard that HQ had admitted that insufficient thought had been given to medical care in this particular offensive. Hayward stood in the courtyard and, everywhere he looked, there were men on stretchers or slumped over on the steps. An entire room had filled up with the amputated arms and legs that were discarded in theatre. He would be happy to confirm to HQ that medical provision was indeed a shambles.

It took a week before the cases were finally cleared. Hayward was exhausted and took himself off for walks in the countryside to clear his mind – and to ready himself for the next onslaught. The CCS would move three more times before November 1918, following the Allied advance to Albert, Brie, Péronne, Roisel and Bellenglise. In his memory, the days would blur into each other. The only day that remained clear was the very first, when he learned the truth about war and what it did to men – the day of his blooding.[18]

5

Wounded

Bert Payne, Montauban, 1 July 1916

I suppose it was worth having the wound, a Blighty to get away
from the Somme. Everyone wanted a Blighty but it depended on
what kind it would be, a good one or a bad one, and mine was
a bad one.

Bert Payne, 1987

The hot coffee that Bert Payne had before going over the top on
the first morning of the Somme would be his last drink for days.
If he'd known, he might have asked for something that tasted
better. The quartermasters who supplied the troops with breakfast
and hot drinks had run out of jugs and urns by the time they got
to Payne's battalion. When they looked around they found thousands of empty fuel cans lying around the supply depots. They
swilled them out as best they could, filled them with coffee and
tea and sent them round to the men. The coffee had a drop of
brandy in it, but even that did little to cover up the lingering
flavour of petrol. Many of the men who hauled themselves up
the trench ladders and died soon afterwards did so with a strange
metallic taste in their mouths. They probably thought it was fear;
in fact it was a mixture of octanes and coffee oils.

Men had been dying for several hours while Payne and his unit
were still waiting for their orders to advance. Payne was leading
a small group of men from the 1st City (Pals') Battalion of the
18th Manchesters. They didn't have to be woken that morning;

they were up and ready to get going. But then no orders had arrived and several hours had passed. An eerie sense of what was happening elsewhere drifted down the line along with the bitter gun smoke. The Pals' excitement began to drain away, leaving behind frustration, bewilderment and fear. To pass the time Payne got his men to play cards and check their wire-cutters, fixing and refixing them to their rifle bayonets, and inspect their little emergency medical kits, which the RMO had given out. The kit wasn't all that impressive. It comprised a cotton dressing with two bandage tails so that it could be tied over and round a wound. Also included was a bottle of iodine so small that it was easily dropped by shaking, muddy soldier fingers when they tried to handle it. It smelled so bad that none of them could imagine ever using it; and, besides, most had forgotten the instructions the doc had given them.

Payne looked at his men, some experienced, others little more than schoolboys. One in particular worried him. He had only been with the battalion for six weeks and he looked as if he wouldn't know what to do with a butter knife, never mind a bayonet. Payne went over to reassure him. Stick close to me, he told the boy. Hang on to me if you have to, lad. With his wide eyes full of terror, the soldier continued to stare at him. Returning to his position at the head of the unit, Payne silently cursed the incompetence of officers who had left the men to stew in their own fear. He had noticed the inferiority of many of his superiors as soon as he arrived at his present posting. The commanding officer had decided to parade the battalion through a town in broad daylight with the band playing, without checking if they were within range of enemy guns. They were, and the results were disastrous. Men were severely wounded as artillery shells smashed down into the parade, and one officer lost both his legs.

Payne was bright, unflappable, with a reputation for good old common sense, so he was soon promoted and made a scout. Scouts were the eyes and ears of the battalion, on whose work lives depended. Payne was good at his job; so good, in fact, that he shot a British officer out for a walk in no-man's-land through the hat when he failed to respond to his hail. By the time of the battle of the Somme, Payne had already saved hundreds of lives. He had found a phoney tree, painted to look like one of the many carcasses left out on the battlefield. But Payne saw it glint oddly in a shaft of sunlight and realised there were German observers hidden inside its canvas and metal frame, sending back instructions to their gunners. Then he had located a pair of seemingly invisible guns hidden in an old railway siding, by working out their bearings from the range of their fire. Bert Payne was a good man to have on your side.

By now a French unit had joined Payne's men and the soldiers were packed up tight against each other. No more card games. Then orders finally came through. They were to take the right-hand flank around the village of Montauban. The target was a small ridge, plain for everyone to see as Payne pointed it out. Then came the shriek of the whistles and Payne led his men over the top. They somehow made it to the first line of enemy trenches and continued to the next one. The schoolboy kept pace with Payne, head down, running for safety, but he was cut down by the machine guns hidden in deep dugouts in the next line of trenches. The practical Payne realised that the Germans must have been preparing themselves for weeks, to appear so quickly in front of them with their equipment set up and ready. Rifles, he just had time to think, were no good; only machine guns were any good. Then he too was cut down, a spray of bullets flying across his face. Falling forward into a shell hole, he saw his teeth fall out of his mouth and hit the ground before he did. All around him, he saw men falling, dead or wounded. They crumpled down around him – one shot through the eyes, another cut open from his jaw to his throat. Then he blacked out.

When he came to in the shell hole, the sky above him was still blue and the sound of the offensive had moved some way off, leaving an eerie silence in the wet mud and among the human debris. Payne gathered himself. He could hear a rasping, guttural sound, like a blocked drain – in-out, in-out. He realised it was his own breathing. That was good, he thought. He must be all right if he could breathe. When he managed to raise himself up on one arm, he couldn't see with his left eye, but the right one was working fine. He got out his field dressing and clamped it down over the closed-up eye, winding the bandage ends around his head. Then he looked at his watch, so precious to a scout and still intact, and saw that it was almost four o'clock. He had been lying unconscious for seven hours. He sat up and looked around. It hurt him to move his head, but he needed to know where he was. Then his eyes met a human face staring back at him, frozen but alive. It was that of his friend Bill Brock, who had been wounded in the foot and was unable to move. He had lain there for hours, waiting for someone else in the shell hole to wake up. He had been watching Payne bleed and twitch, fearful that he would die. They were the only survivors.

Payne crawled over to Brock and told him, through his ragged lips and cheeks, that they would be heading back. Brock tried to shake off the horrible sight of Payne's face and pointed to his foot: a tattered little shock of pink and bloody flesh in the brown mud. It had all but been shot off and, although he had managed to get his boot off to relieve the pain, there was no way he could walk. Payne was having none of it. He took his friend's field dressing and tied the foot up as best he could. Then he slowly put Brock's boot back on, quietly reassuring him when the other man cried out in pain and begged him to stop. Payne laced the boot up to support Brock's foot and then looked around for a spare rifle to use as a crutch. If they didn't leave now, they would die in the shell hole. Brock knew it was useless to argue with the scout, so he scrambled up somehow and leaned on the rifle.

Together they clambered out of the crater – one man limping, trying to find a painless way to walk, leaning on a dead man's rifle; the other with his bandaged eye and ragged face – willing each other on, to a chorus of distant gunfire: the half-blind leading the lame. The landscape they had viewed from the forward trench that morning had almost totally disappeared, churned up like a building site, an obstacle course of collapsed trenches and shell holes. Dropping down into one trench, they found much to their surprise the regimental chaplain and one of the RMOs, heading for the front line. They were both good men, by Payne's book, and had become inseparable – the padre supporting the doctor when he needed help, and the doctor helping the padre with the communion service that he held at a drumhead behind the lines. But what were they doing here? Showing his disregard for rank, Payne let rip with a stream of swearing. They must go back to the dressing station, where they were needed. They shouldn't be here, where everybody was dead. They were likely to be killed pointlessly, when there were so many men who needed them to stay alive. And no, he didn't need any help: he could walk, and Brock was doing well with his crutch. They'd get back in their own time or find a bearer on the way.

But there weren't any bearers. So many had been killed in the first few hours of the offensive that RMOs at the aid posts refused to let any more bearers out on to the field. Payne and Brock were on their own among the dead, struggling to make their way out. A few hundred yards further on they stopped to rest in a shell hole, where they found a man almost blown to pieces, but somehow still alive. He was gasping for air, sobbing and calling out for someone called Annie. Payne could see at a glance that there was no hope for the man: he was bound to die after hours of lonely agony. Payne took up the rifle Brock was using as a crutch and shot the soldier. Then he and Brock moved on in silence. He deserved a VC, Payne thought, for the courage that spared a man such a horrible death.

By now enemy guns were roaring at the British lines and the two men found themselves in the line of fire. They got knocked off their feet and fell down into a shell hole full of barbed wire. But they got up and continued their journey, their ears ringing, their hands and faces scratched, and Payne's breeches ripped to pieces at the back. When they finally reached their own lines it was hard to recognise the organised trench network they had left that morning. Instead they found chaos, with trenches no longer connected to one another, but full of wounded or confused men and abandoned equipment. Climbing down into one trench, they found it full of POWs, bound and guarded by sentries. By now Brock was in so much pain that he was sobbing, tears running down his cheeks. But there was no one to help him here. One of the sentries pointed to a place in the distance where he believed there was a medical post.

When they finally got to the place, not only did they find a medical post, but a horse-drawn ambulance preparing to leave. It was full up with injured German POWs, but by that time Payne no longer cared. He tipped enough men off their stretchers to make space for his wounded friend, leaving them on the roadside calling for help. Then he loaded up Brock and called for the driver to set out. Shortly afterwards he found another ambulance and got on himself. As it bumped along, Payne watched walking wounded and carts full of dead moving in one direction and reinforcements rushing the other way. Montauban had been captured, he heard – one of the few successes of the day – although it wasn't to be held. If he squinted, he could still make out the village with his undamaged eye, but it gradually disappeared into the distance as he bumped down the track, listening to the swish of the horse's tail, its occasional snorts and his own slurping breath.

The ambulance finally stopped at a medical station at Abbeville, where Payne was helped down and onto a stretcher. For the first time since he had come to the war, he was no longer upright and self-reliant, just one of hundreds of casualties lying outside the medical officers' tents, helpless and waiting. He could hear orderlies selecting men on stretchers for treatment at the post. Then more ambulances pulled up, horse-drawn and motorised, and a few wounded would be loaded onto them for the next stage of their journey. But none of this seemed to reduce the numbers of men lying unattended outside the tents. Payne tried to sleep and ignore the cries of the dying all around him.

The next day was worse. Where there had been numbness in his face, there was now horrible pain. His cheeks and tongue had swollen up so that he could no longer make himself understood. Payne, who had always prided himself on his initiative and independence, had become helpless. He was moved inside the post and as the day passed he watched the doctors and bearers struggle with the hundreds of wounded and dying men. The whole medical system had collapsed under the weight of the Somme's casualties and pinned him to the spot. But at least he wouldn't get typhus or tetanus: he had been inoculated three times that day. Each time an orderly came forward with a syringe he had tried to tell him that he had already had the shot, but the man couldn't understand him and gave him another injection. When he tried to point at his casualty label so that they would at least update it, he noticed that he hadn't been given one.

So he lay and waited, the pain growing along with a terrible thirst. He'd had nothing since breakfast coffee in the forward trenches the previous day, and now he couldn't ask for a drink. Even if he could, the orderly would have been hard pressed to get liquid past the rags of his face. His dressings were changed a couple of times but nothing more. Then he felt his stretcher bump and rise. An exhausted bearer appeared over him and told him he was being moved to the train station and that he was going home. Payne was too tired and diminished to care.

On board the train he saw that the staff were coping no better than those at the medical post. The trains specially designed to transport the wounded had been filled and had left days ago. Now only the most basic rolling stock was left, with no berths for stretchers or cushions or kitchens, just hard wooden seats, few lavatories and even fewer medical personnel. The journey to the coast took four days. Payne thought it might have been quicker to walk. He lay while they had to wait endlessly in sidings and at crossroads to let pass supply trains full of reinforcements and ammunition. And still no one was feeding him or giving him water; all they did was push a morphine tablet onto his tongue

6

Nurses

Jentie Patterson, Winifred Kenyon, Elizabeth Boon

As a patient I would rather have a good nurse than a good physician. A physician gives his blessing, the surgeon does the operation. But it is the nurse who does the work.

Henry Souttar, *No. 1 Belgian Field Hospital*[1]

One night in her office at the No. 5 Casualty Clearing Station on
the Normandy coast, Sister Jentie Patterson set aside the last of
her official paperwork and started a letter to her sister Martha in
Scotland. Even though she was exhausted and a cold wind had
found its way through the wooden planks of her hut and had
frozen her hands and feet to numbness, she hadn't written for a
long time and felt it couldn't wait another day. So she lit a candle,
wrapped herself in blankets, put her feet on her ceramic hot-water
bottle under her chair and started to write. When she had finished,
she was amazed to find that two hours had gone by, her candle
had burned to a nub and she had poured out all her feelings about
her new post and her new life. It was late November 1914.

No. 5 CCS had been set up just outside Tréport to process
casualties coming from the front to the hospital ships on the
Channel coast. It was an abandoned monastery, with dormitories
and some tenting that served as extra ward space. Like all CCSs
in 1914, it was intended as a staging post, where dressings were
changed and fluids administered before the men were moved on
to their next destination. But in 'the race to the sea' the German

so that his pain was controlled, after a fashion. The train pushed on so slowly it felt as if it was being dragged, just as he had dragged Bill Brock across the torn landscape of the battlefield.

But even when the train finally stopped at Le Havre, Payne's journey was far from over. The hospital ship, the SS *Saltaire*, ran with fair efficiency, but there were rumours of submarines, so it stayed in the harbour all night before setting sail. By now, drugged and dehydrated, Payne was punch-drunk from the suffering all around him. A glance in a dirty train window had shown him his swollen, bandaged face and for the first time in his life he felt he had no idea what the future might hold for him. He slept whenever he could. At the station in England he tried once again to tell someone he was thirsty, already knowing that there would be no point. Yet this time, almost miraculously, he made himself understood. One of the ladies receiving the trains appraised him with a practical eye and whirled away. She returned with a teapot and a bowl of sugar. Payne indicated that yes, he took sugar, so she stirred several spoonfuls straight into the pot and then manoeuvred the spout carefully into the least-damaged part of Payne's mouth. It was his first drink for days, standing on the platform of a British railway station, hope suddenly visible somewhere in the distance.

armies tried to outflank the Allies, and now No. 5 was in the thick of it, the furthest medical facility up the line. Sister Patterson could hear the guns roar day and night and she knew it meant they weren't just a staging post any more.

It hadn't been a promising start at the CCS when she arrived. The colonel in command had made it pretty clear that he hadn't wanted female nurses at his station. In his opinion, there was no place for women in France. Yet when they had to care for the first wave of more than 200 casualties he hadn't apologised exactly, but he'd gone round congratulating the nurses afterwards, admitting that he didn't know what he would have done without them. Patterson had worked at a general hospital in Versailles, which ran on similar lines to the large metropolitan hospitals back in Britain – formal, planned, organised. In fact, that was the reason she left. It was all a bit too much like nursing at home. She had wanted the challenge of working close to the front, and now she had got it.

At No. 5 she could no longer distinguish between nursing and informed improvisation. There were no shifts, just more work than she would ever have thought possible. On their first 200-patient day, almost all the casualties were on stretchers. The men were too embarrassed to let the nurses undress them, as most were riddled with lice, so the orderlies were needed everywhere at once. They wouldn't even let the nurses take their boots and socks off, so bad was the state of their trench feet. But the nurses stayed with them until late into the night, when the last ambulance pulled away to take the wounded to the base hospital. Then at last they retired to their dormitories, all of them in agony with backache from nursing bent double over the low stretchers.

The next day, with two hours' notice, 300 new casualties arrived. By evening they were cleaned and fed and stabilised and ready to move on. The nurses waited up with their patients, but midnight came and went and still no ambulances arrived to take them away. Then they heard that no ambulances would be coming, so the wounded had to stay overnight, no matter that the CCS hadn't been designed for that. Inside the tented wards there were no beds, sheets or pillows, only stretchers. Sister Patterson and her nurses had to use all their skill and ingenuity to make the men comfortable. They found straw and blankets, and rolled up spare aprons and towels as pillows. They had no pyjamas, either, so the men had to sleep in their uniforms to keep warm, which meant doing the fastest laundry round on record the next morning. And they only had tea and cocoa for one serving per day, so they made that last as long as possible.

All the while the little operating theatre they had converted from a side room was working around the clock. They were dealing with head injuries, abdominal wounds, bad fractures with smashed bones and ragged veins. Many lives were lost on the operating table, but more men came out alive than dead. Sister Patterson realised that it didn't take a fully equipped base hospital to save a badly wounded man's life. But you couldn't do without nurses.

And you needed nurses with some gumption – the ability just to get on with it. Women who weren't too conventional. Take the CCS's neatly arranged, full-to-capacity store cupboards, for instance: they'd been scrapped after the second day. Instead, the nurses had got together all the buckets they could find and filled each of them with a selection of dressings, bandages, morphine, scissors and cloths, then lined them up along the wall of the receiving hall. As they escorted the men through to their wards, the nurses could just grab a bucket with the essential equipment, without having to run back and forth to the store cupboard and fill out the supply forms. It was such a good idea that the surgeons soon did the same. Their buckets joined the ones along the wall, filled with swabs and surgical scrubs and instruments, so that they could take one as they followed a patient who urgently needed surgery. Sister Patterson rather liked the look of those buckets. They seemed to symbolise the new type of hospital that No. 5 was becoming: a place where the staff responded quickly, thought on their feet, saved lives.

The windows of her little hut rattled. It wasn't the wind; it was the guns, still going hard. She wouldn't get much sleep tonight. Sister Patterson finished her letter. She was pleased with how well she had been able to describe her experience, and with how much she was coming to understand.

On 7 December they took in 300 wounded at one o'clock. Fortunately this time enough ambulances had arrived to take away most of them by supper time, but twenty were left, and they were all in a bad way, so each man was looked after by a nurse all night. The days that followed were quiet. The twenty patients were stable and Sister Patterson got to know them. One of them had been wounded at the first battle of Ypres and had been shuttling around various aid posts before arriving at No. 5, where the surgeons had finally put him right. He was relieved to be on his way home and grateful for the good care. He even gave Sister Patterson an elaborate belt buckle that he had taken off a Prussian. She talked to him about the war and the soldier told her she needed to visit the front line herself, if she really wanted to understand what was going on. So she found an orderly to accompany her and together they hopped into an ambulance that was on its way to the trenches. There she saw for herself how cold it was and why her patients' feet were in such a bad state. She saw what rations they were on and why so many arrived hungry. She saw how filthy the conditions were, the mud and the stink. She saw the daily struggle for survival in the trenches and out on the battlefield. And she saw how CCS No. 5 was part of that war.

Back at home in Scotland, Martha was proving to be just as capable as her sister. In response to her sister's letter she had mobilised the local community, and now regular supply parcels were arriving at No. 5. There were large quantities of soap, for washing people and floors. And the knitters were off: the women had taken out their needles and yarn when Martha read them her sister's letter, and now they were knitting socks and scarves for the patients. One day Sister Patterson gave out 200 pairs of socks and she never missed an opportunity to encourage more from Martha. She wished everyone would be as efficient as her sister.

At the CCS the colonel continued to make a fat ass of himself. He was fine at giving the orders, but most of the time he got them wrong. Like most doctors, he didn't have the patience or the attention to detail that was needed for effective nursing. All the nurses had found themselves saving his reputation more than once. It was difficult not to heckle when he made a patriotic speech during a dinner held for the nurses in the New Year.

January 1915 was extremely cold and Jentie got bad chilblains all over her feet. They had received a visit from a specialist who gave them a series of lectures on how to look after the feet of men with frostbite, trench foot or marching injuries. He told them to dress them only lightly and, where possible, to get them aired. Sister Patterson had attended a massage therapy course, so the specialist showed her how to adapt her knowledge to the special needs of soldiers' feet. He warned her that, from now on, she would never be without work. The nurses started paying attention to their own needs as well, asking their families to send them wellington boots to protect their feet as they rushed along the muddy paths between the long, tented wards that were now a permanent fixture at No. 5.

The cold continued well into March. The colonel summoned all his senior staff to warn them that battle was about to be rejoined, at Neuve Chapelle, later that month. They would be one of the hospitals receiving and treating casualties in the new tented wards. None of them needed telling. They had all noticed the increase in traffic on the roads. But there was some good news too: they were to be sent equipment for an extra eighty-eight beds. The delivery lorries brought the mattresses only to the front door, so the nurses spent all day dragging them up steps and through corridors, along the muddy paths and into the wards. It was exhausting, but at least they now had proper beds. There would be no more back-breaking days bent over stretchers.

The battle began on 10 March and they got their first casualties that evening. On the second day the hospital's well gave out, and by evening they were seriously short of water. On the third day

Sister Patterson found herself almost overwhelmed by the weight of it all, so she went for a short walk into the woods nearby. When she heard a lark, it brought a smile to her face. She realised that she hadn't smiled since the first ambulance full of shattered soldiers had pulled up three days before. She decided she would smile as much as she could from now on. She would try to be cheery, both for the sake of the wounded men and for herself. On the evening of the fourth day the nurses attended a short service, during which they sang the hymn 'Peace, Perfect Peace'. Not much of that, Sister Patterson thought. After the service the colonel congratulated them on how well they had coped with the first wave of patients. They knew what that meant: there was about to be a second wave.

There was a couple of days' breathing space, during which they mended the well and cleaned the wards. Then the second wave of Neuve Chapelle casualties arrived. Fifteen of them were suffering from enteric conditions, the like of which Sister Patterson had never seen before, and one of the tented wards was quickly converted into a special enteric block. What must it have been like for them out there, in the mud and filth, she thought. They were still receiving patients at the end of March. These were the worst casualties of all: some had lain on the battlefield for days and their wounds were rank and rotting. Most of them were unable to speak, so the staff had to work out what was wrong with them from their ticket, if they were lucky, or by guesswork. Many came in with high fevers, and all of them had to be nursed constantly to keep them alive. Patterson had one soldier to care for who had the highest fever she had ever experienced in her professional life – 105.4 degrees Fahrenheit. Saving his life became her way of fighting back against it all. She sat with him all through the night. By the morning his temperature was slightly down and it continued to fall, little by little, all day. He would survive.

That day Sister Patterson was put in charge of one of the extra surgical wards that had been set up in the new tents. It had 100 beds, three nurses, five orderlies, and every single bed contained an acute case. Despite having been up all night with her fever patient, she worked for twelve hours straight. When someone finally came to relieve her, she stood for a moment at the tent entrance and looked back at her ward. She didn't feel much satisfaction or pride. After twelve hours she hadn't even been able to see all the patients. But before it all threatened to become unbearable again, she set off for another walk in the woods. Spring had arrived and everywhere she looked there were bright-green and yellow daffodils poking through the undergrowth. She started to pick them – and the time passed softly, until she had picked enough for all the wards. When she returned she found all the spare jugs they had and set the daffodils out on tables: a little sunshine brought in from the woods.

In April a specialist surgeon arrived to open an eye ward at No. 5. Sister Patterson spent as much time there as she could, learning from him. When she wrote to Martha now, she marvelled at how expert they had all become. One day they had taken in 103 cases in mid-morning and by 5 p.m. all the patients were admitted and comfortable. It was almost satisfying. And they did it with an ever-changing staff. Other CCSs were always asking No. 5 to loan them their expert nurses, so they were usually short-handed. The new nurses who arrived on a monthly basis took a lot of training to get up to speed and often they weren't worth much in the first couple of days, when their immunisations made them tired. Sister Patterson was almost always an orderly or two short as well. When she looked at her letters to her sister, she saw that she was constantly grumbling – about lazy orderlies, convoys arriving at half an hour's notice, ambulances coming to collect patients in the middle of the night. She hoped Martha didn't mind, but she tried never to let the patients see how she really felt. With Martha's support, and the quiet hope of the woods, she could go on with the work of the war.

When Winifred Kenyon applied for nursing service in France, she never considered going anywhere else but a casualty clearing station. She wanted to be as close to the war as possible, to share in the adventure and excitement and to make her contribution. She wanted to nurse – really nurse – not mop floors and take orders all day. A friend had told her that most of the CCSs were in fields, with grass or canvas for floors; not much mopping needed there. When her posting came through in the late summer of 1915, it was just what she had hoped for: she would be sent to a casualty clearing station for serious cases behind the front at Verdun. It meant a long lorry hop from the French coast, changing transport several times in towns and army camps.

The driver of the last lorry swore he was going to take her right up to the front door of the CCS, but as they pushed deeper and deeper into the countryside, Kenyon began to worry. Surely there couldn't possibly be a hospital out here, in the fields and woods, hours away from any towns or villages? Then the road turned and headed straight for a wood. In the distance she could see yards of washing hung out on a line that disappeared into the trees. That must be it, Kenyon thought, and it's laundry day. As they got closer she realised that these weren't linen sheets, but row upon row of white canvas tents stretching in and around the wood. They had arrived at the casualty clearing station, right there in the middle of nowhere. The lorry pushed along a gravelled track and stopped in a circular driveway. There were tents all around it and a huge signpost, with arrows pointing every which way. It was, as the driver had promised, the front door. Kenyon jumped down, thanked him and went over to the signpost, looking for the arrow showing the way to the nurses' quarters. It seemed like the sensible place to start.

It was a long way to the nurses' quarters and, on the way, Kenyon looked around her new home. She had never worked in a hospital where you looked up to see the sky instead of the ceiling as you walked between wards. As she passed nurses darting in and out of the tents, she knew how much she would have to learn from them, to get used to this strange new world. Then, as her first weeks and months at the CCS slipped by and she became one of those nurses darting between tents, she realised that there was just as much to learn outside the wards – basic things that didn't require a nursing exam, but were every bit as fundamental to her work.

Take the weather, for instance. Weather dominated the lives of the men and women working at CCSs on the windswept plains of France. The wide-open landscape looked wonderful in the sunshine, but when the wind blew, it blew hard, and it blew almost all year round. Nurses got used to the sound of the canvas tents buffeting in the wind wherever they worked. CCS tents were firmly pegged down, so it sounded worse than it was, but now and again cyclones ripped down rows of tents, injuring the men in their beds all over again and terrifying everyone with their destructive power.[2]

When winter came, all the nurses had their families send extra woollens. As the temperature dropped, they gave up on night-wear and slept in their uniforms and multiple layers of socks to keep warm. There was always a sturdy stove in their quarters, which they kept going all night. Sometimes when the nurses came on duty in the morning it was red-hot and you had to be careful not to start the day with a nasty burn from brushing past it. Hot-water bottles were the best, pushed down the bottom of a camp bed to banish the damp, although there were never enough to go round. Then there were the nights when every-thing in the entire CCS would freeze: milk, butter, cooking oil, ink – even the chilblain lotion. Everyone gathered round the stoves, wrapped in all the clothes they could find, and waited for their world to thaw.[3]

Whatever time of year it was, rain always meant trouble. The paths between the tents became swamps, boots got stuck in the mud, and if they tripped, that was it for their clean uniforms. Pushing trolleys along the paths was almost impossible, so everyone waited until the rain cleared up before moving patients from one ward to another. In some places it rained for weeks on end, and nurses gave up trying to stay dry and clean. One made herself a waterproof uniform skirt out of tarpaulin, another mended a hole in her tent roof by pushing an umbrella through the vent and opening it up; it worked, so they left it until the summer before patching up the roof.[4] Rain also created a great deal of extra work in the wards themselves. Rain at the front meant mud, and mud meant long carries, trench foot and infection.[5] Trenchfoot, Kenyon would learn, was a wound inflicted by the battlefield itself. It could bring a man down as hard and long as a bit of shrapnel and could take just as much effort to nurse.

Most nurses thought about the weather as soon as they woke up and listened, to guess what the day would bring. If there was no sound of wind buffeting their tent, or rain drumming on the canvas, it might be a good day to do the laundry themselves rather than send it into town. If there was a river nearby, doing the laundry could be fun in the summer, all the nurses rolling up their uniform sleeves, laughing and chatting as an infinite number of sheets were pegged to infinite lengths of washing line. There was so much laundry to do, with some men needing a change of bedclothes several times a day, that it could be disheartening. But then the nurses remembered how much their patients appreciated the luxury of clean linen – a fresh sheet, a white pillow case, fluffed blankets – so they scrubbed and pegged and folded, understanding that this too was an act of nursing and healing.[6]

Perhaps the most unexpected thing Kenyon learned inside the ward tents was how much was left up to the nurses themselves. There were several wards that they ran without doctors, and they taught their skills to the new arrivals like Kenyon. 'Resus' was one of them. The men there were too weak to raise their heads, let alone be operated on, and it was the nurses who brought them back from the brink. Kenyon learned to administer the magic mixtures of hot saline, brandy and coffee, and that you could never have too many hot-water bottles. Sometimes you put ten or twelve around a man close to death from hypothermia and gradually watched him come back to life. Men came in grey and went out pink. The first time a surgeon congratulated her on saving a man's life and making it possible for him to operate, she was delighted. Then she did it again, and then every day after that. Eventually it didn't seem like anything at all.

Kenyon was pleased to have started her work in the resus ward. She felt she was making an immediate contribution. And it was such a good place to learn. While she waited for her patient to revive, she asked the other nurses about the entries on the casualty tickets. She could work out some of what the MO back at the aid post had written, but some of the acronyms were new to her. 'ICT', for instance, stood for 'I Can't Tell' – it was the MO's way of saying that the man was so badly injured that he couldn't work out what needed doing first. What it really meant was: 'Nurse, sort it out, please, and come and get a surgeon when the patient is stable.'[7] Then there was 'SI' and 'DI' – 'Severely Ill' and 'Dangerously Ill'. These patients might be warmed up and rehydrated in resus, but as soon as they were stable they were brought to the moribund ward.

Studying tickets was a really good way to learn about the nuts and bolts of casualty. Kenyon thought what a good system it was: one bit of paper that stayed with you all the way to the hospital or home. It was good until it failed. If you lost your ticket, that meant all manner of trouble. You could end up in the wrong place, getting treatment for the wrong condition, or simply end up getting ignored. People had died for want of a ticket. And it was good until someone wrote it up incorrectly. That was something all the nurses knew: whatever you do, don't let doctors write up tickets unsupervised, especially tickets for patients going on the ambulance trains. All they do is write what operations the man has had. They don't fill in any of the really useful information, like the diet and drinks required, and whether the patient can sit or lie. And they never remember to mark the ticket with the big red X that means the patient has to be given twenty-four-hour care, if he is to survive the journey.

Doctors, Kenyon soon concluded, were all very well, but without nurses there wasn't really any point even pitching the tents. Inside the long canvas wards she walked for miles each day, checking charts, giving out medication, changing dressings and linen.[8] She had to be alert to the slightest change in her patient – his colour, his breathing, his temperature – and then take the decision about whether to call a busy surgeon. It was also worth knowing how full her wards were going to be in the days to come. She learned that the best people to ask about that were the ambulance drivers. They were the only people at the front who had any idea about what was really going on.[9]

Then there was the kind of work she hadn't been trained for before she came to France. It was nurses who waited for a young soldier to wake up from an operation so that they could console him when he realised that his legs had been amputated.[10] It was nurses who held the hand of a man whilst they guided him to a mirror so that he could see for the first time his empty pyjama sleeve, neatly folded and pinned up high where he had lost his arm. They carried a good supply of handkerchiefs at all times. Men cried in their arms until the fronts of their aprons were wet. And while a man cried, the nurses discreetly looked about the ward to see what else needing doing – where pillows had fallen or blankets had got tangled around broken limbs; who needed a drink or salve on dry chapped lips; who needed a smile and some reassurance. Kenyon was surprised at how quickly she got used to the gentle, comforting lie. Yes, you will get better. No one at home has forgotten you. Anaesthetics really aren't that bad. Everything will be all right. The war won't go on for ever – or at least, it can't possibly get any worse.

She stopped telling that lie in the summer of 1916. The CCS was full to bursting by the end of the first day of the Somme offensive. It was sunny and warm, so they could at least leave the sides of the tents open, but the heat had caused some men to be baked in carapaces of mud from the battlefield.[11] Inside the receiving tent, one nurse and an orderly spent the whole of the first week just chipping off mud. Sister called a quick meeting in the mess: they couldn't break, no matter what. The men who had managed to survive long enough to get here depended on them. Don't let them see you cry, whatever happens. So Kenyon greeted each soldier who arrived, whether he could hear it or not, with a cheery 'Good morning' or 'Good afternoon'. There wasn't much time for telling lies, but she smiled all day long until that, too, felt like lying.[12]

Normal duties and postings were ignored for the first weeks of the Somme offensive. Everyone did what they needed to do. Kenyon went into the kitchen once and found an MO making sandwiches and coffee, because everyone in his ward was starving but too busy – and he was the only one not needed at that precise moment. In another ward the chaplain was shaving patients who were going for surgery. One of the men winked at a nurse and asked what sort of tip she thought he ought to give the padre. Suddenly the entire ward was convulsed with laughter.[13]

Kenyon saw the staff working together more closely than ever before. They worked as one, desperate to save lives, and crushed when they failed. They were so close to the front that they felt part of it, fighting alongside the soldiers. But their work was taking its toll. It was boiling hot, and their uniforms stuck to their bodies, clammy with sweat and dirt.[14] No one was getting enough to eat or drink. By the fourth day Kenyon knew she couldn't go on and tried to find a quiet bed in the nurses' quarters. When she collapsed, still dressed, she had difficulty going to sleep, with the day's events racing through her head. But then she thought of how they had survived and held their part of the line. There was satisfaction in that. Then she fell asleep.

It hadn't been like that everywhere. Into the second week of the offensive, Kenyon heard from friends at other CCSs who had simply been overwhelmed by patients. One nurse wrote that it had been like Scutari. She had done twenty-four stretches of theatre duty in two weeks and it had nearly defeated her.[15] Another noticed a sudden lack of abdominal cases coming into the moribund ward and suspected that RMOs were leaving them as moribund at the aid posts, so as not to swamp the CCSs with yet more desperate cases.[16] But there was no stemming the tide. From another CCS came stories of how hundreds and hundreds of men on stretchers had simply been abandoned outside their tents, with little hope that the staff would get to all those who lay there. Instead the nurses made up little packages of morphine and dressings and handed them to the men on stretchers each time they rushed past them on their way from one ward to another, leaving them to treat themselves. It would be days before all of them could be seen by a nurse, and over a week before a bed was found for the last of the survivors. By then many had died, their bodies tipped onto the ground by bearers desperate for stretchers. Kenyon understood why nurses were always running in CCSs that were overwhelmed by the influx of patients: it was not just because they were needed everywhere at once, but because they couldn't bear to stop.

By late autumn of 1916 the last of the Somme's wounded were quietly recovering in the wards or being put on trains bound for Britain. Slowly the CCSs returned to normal. At last the nurses had time to gather in the evening in one of the dormitory tents to laugh at each other's dressing gowns and slippers and to swap stories. Kenyon found that she had missed this time for friendship and laughter more than anything else during the summer.[17] This was when they nursed each other. They made rounds of cocoa and read out their letters, telling each other about their families and their lives at home. They reminded each other to eat properly, because life in the fresh air made them ravenous. They shared their food parcels, and when Kenyon got sent a simnel cake they threw a party in its honour, toasting it with mugs of cocoa and finishing it to the last crumb on the greaseproof-paper wrapping. If they had the energy and sufficient light, the nurses sewed while they talked, mending stockings and tears on their uniforms and sewing buttons on shirts.

There was still some excitement, even after their sector had eventually gone quiet. Nurses visited the battlefield and brought back reports of tanks and piles of shells wherever you looked.

Then, one night, a Zeppelin was shot down right over their wood. All the staff rushed out to watch it burst into flames and slowly drop through the sky, before crashing to the ground. Kenyon got as close as she could and grabbed pieces of twisted aluminium as souvenirs, wrapping them in her apron. She passed the fragments around her ward, still warm from the fire, and the patients wanted to hear every detail of the crash. Kenyon was always amazed at how fascinated soldiers were with mementos of the war. Heaven forbid that the surgeon should forget to save any bits of shrapnel that he'd dug out of them. They wanted to keep them, wrapped in a bit of bandage, pinned to their pillow.

Seeing the remains of the Zeppelin every morning reminded Kenyon that they were closer to the war than to any town or other human habitation. Yet working so closely together and relying on each other, they never felt isolated, and they had created supply lines of their own – long and thin, but resilient – stretching all the way home.[18] They all had their sewing circle or community group.[19] Kenyon's group had excellent knitters, but there were others who ensured that the CCS never ran out of pyjamas or pillow cases, scarves or socks. One of the simplest but most important things they needed from home were the linen drawstring bags for the men to store their possessions in. Often a casualty had nothing left but what he carried when he was wounded, and these few things were precious to him. When men came round in the ward, nurses would show them how they had gathered up their things and put them in a bag hanging securely on their bed.

One day, instead of drawstring bags, they received a whole box of tiny lavender bags. They wondered for a while what to do with them, before taking them to their wards.[20] There were men whose injuries were rank, despite their best efforts, and the nurses gave them the little bags to hold and sniff, or pinned them to their pillow or sheets. The smell masked the gangrene and the rot, and the scent calmed them and reminded them of home. Farms in Norfolk produced plenty of lavender, so there was no shortage, and the nurses soon requested more.

The period of quiet gave Kenyon and her colleagues time to spend with individual patients. She could see them becoming more stable or recovering, eventually going home or returning to the front line. She wasn't just looking out for changes in pallor or temperature, she also observed changes to their mood. She noticed who was getting bored or frustrated, and went to look for magazines or books for them. When the rain drummed on the canvas roof, driving some of the patients mad, nurses tried to find a gramophone to play some music that would drown out the sound.[21]

When mail came, Kenyon noticed that it wasn't greeted with the same excitement by everyone. Some patients were cast down by news from home that told of hardship and penury, children without Christmas presents, wives with no money left at the end of the week. Kenyon and some other nurses got together to raise money for these families. They contacted local charities in the patient's home town or village and asked them to check up on his family and pass on their donations. Thus they often caught families who had slipped through the net of larger organisations dedicated to the welfare of soldiers' kin. Nursing beyond the front, they got families back on their feet from a distance, while they restored their loved ones in their wards.

For Kenyon and the other nurses, the CCS in the wood became a little world of its own. They even spent their off-duty hours around the place: it was too far to travel to a town unless you were staying away for a week or so. So they improvised and created their own entertainment. They borrowed some of the staff officers' horses and went riding; others went for long walks and got to know the local flora and fauna. Kenyon marked time in the CCS by the natural cyles in the woods: the falling of leaves, the hibernation of the squirrels, the green shoots poking through the moss. Sometimes, when they had only half an hour's break, the nurses would stand quietly to work out where the sound of the guns was coming from. Then they would head off in the opposite direction, just far enough for there to be silence.[22]

There they sat while the minutes passed, soft and soundless. Then they got up, brushed off their skirts and returned to work.

Christmas 1916 was celebrated with particular abandon at the CCS. The nurses cooked Christmas puddings for the entire station, using enamel chamber pots. They were the perfect size, and and Kenyon wondered if it would ever catch on at home. It had been quiet in their part of the line and everyone was looking forward to the celebration. Decorating their wards was essential. There would be not a stick of holly or train of ivy left in the wood after the nurses had been through it, and anything that would do as a Christmas tree was dug and potted up. They had even found some mistletoe, and the men became almost hysterical with joy when they hung up a bunch in their ward. In their turn, the patients made enough paper chains to stretch from there to the coast. Kenyon had sown some forget-me-not seeds in the spring and she had pressed the flowers so that the men could put them inside the cards they were sending home.

Any excuse for a party was good enough. The nurses most enjoyed fancy-dress parties and paraded their costumes in front of the patients in the ward so that they could judge which was best. Probably the most inspired entry anywhere on the front was that of the nurse who went as 'A Blighty Case', a patient who would be returning to England.[23] She wrapped herself in an army greatcoat and scarf, bandaged up both legs and arms and her head, and put on a pair of the felt slippers that were given to men with bad trench foot. Then she mocked up a huge 'Blighty ticket', properly filled out and tied to the button of the coat. When she entered the ward and skated up and down in her huge slippers, the men cheered and clapped enough to raise the canvas roof. She took bow after bow, before inevitably being awarded the Best in Show prize.

Nurses, like bearers, kept pets under any circumstances. Most CCSs attracted a troop of sturdy dogs and cats that had been abandoned in the smashed French towns and villages. Kenyon's CCS had two fox cubs, Satan and Prince. Prince had rickets and very bandy back legs. You could spot him a mile off with his odd little gait, shambling down the path to the bins at the back of the kitchen tent. The foxes were joined by the posh French hunting dog rescued by the chief surgeon, and they all paid their way at the CCS by patrolling the food stores and keeping down the rat population. But that wasn't all they were good for. Kenyon struggled to get patients up and walking once they had recovered sufficiently, but asking them to walk the animals always got them out of bed. And usually after that they looked for other little jobs to pass the hours, so Kenyon got them to do the ironing and boot-polishing that took up so much of her time, or filling up hot-water bottles from saucepans on the ward stove. When they were stronger they helped the bearers to move patients around the ward – although the sight of it also made Kenyon feel sad: if they were able to do that, then they would soon be strong enough to return to the front line.

By 1917 the wards were becoming very well organised. There were bridge tournaments, chess games, concerts and a library trolley. They played netball on the short court marked out at the limits of the CCS, and created a league whose results were followed by all the patients. Sometimes there was so much to do off-duty, Kenyon wondered how they would cope when the offensives began again. Their favourite game was a paperchase, which became the high point of the summer weekends. Staff checked the weather forecast and tried to find out if there would be fighting nearby. If it looked as if there would be a clear, warm and peaceful day, plans went ahead.

On game day, nurses and doctors divided themselves into teams: the Hares and the Hounds; Kenyon was usually a Hare. Everyone who could be moved out of the wards gathered around the start and finish line just outside the station, some standing, others sitting in chairs or lying on stretchers. Over the previous days the patients had ripped old newspaper into small pieces and loaded them into borrowed bearer-panniers. Now each Hare was given a satchel of paper and ran off into the forest, throwing out a trail of paper behind them. Each followed a separate route and, after

a set time, the chief surgeon blew a whistle, restrained the dog
and foxes, and set the Hounds team after the Hares. The Hounds
had to find each individual Hare and march them back over the
finish line. The winner was the last Hound or Hare to come in.

The game lasted for hours, sometimes a whole sunny day and
into the evening, and the men cheered each time a player was
finally brought home. Kenyon was good at the game, eluding
capture for hours, and finally getting back to the finish line
exhausted and with her muscles aching from all the running. But
it made her so happy. As she waited to see who would come in
next, she watched the patients cheering in their pyjamas and
tunics, laughing, pointing and taking surreptitious bets; and in
the wood, young nurses and doctors were darting in and out of
the trees, full of laughter and fun. For a time it seemed that was
all there was. No CCS, no war, just the wood and the game and
the joy it brought. Both Hares and Hounds would limp for days,
but it was worth it.

One evening, after a long game, Kenyon wrote home to her
family about the day and how she had ended up being the winning
Hare. She told them how beautiful the woods could be in summer,
and how uplifted she was to hear the cheers of men she tended
every day following her through the sunshine, drowning out the
distant guns. Her family was horrified. Surely she was not at the
CCS to have fun, they replied. She was there on serious business,
to nurse the wounded in a war that she was clearly taking far too
lightly. They didn't understand, but Kenyon wasn't angry with
them. In her next letter home she simply wrote that she wished
there would be many more games and a lot less war.

Nurse Elizabeth Boon sat up late one night catching up on her
correspondence. It was November 1918, four years almost to the
day since Jentie Patterson stayed up to write to her sister Martha.
The war had finally come to an end. But Nurse Boon's hadn't
finished: she still had a letter to write.

Dear Mrs Simpson

You will have heard the sad news that your son Pte Joseph Simpson passed away on Tuesday November 12th. The funeral is taking place today at Terlincthun Cemetary. The No. of his grave is 4E Plat 10. We would have liked to have you with him but when we saw he was so acutely ill there was no time to get you here before he died. He passed away peacefully at 5.52 on Tuesday 12th November.

He talked of going to Blighty to see you and then before he died he thought he was with you all and put out his hands to first one and then the other with such a glad smile, he called you by name and then 'Ada' but we could not catch what else he said. He was a very good patient and we did all we could for him and he had everything that was possible.

With sincere sympathy

E. Boon

(for Matron)

Boon worked on the moribund ward at her CCS. Moribund wards – the last stop at the CCS for those soldiers beyond help – had been given their own RAMC regulations, and it was according to regulation that special care was taken to safeguard the belongings of the dying, and that the patient's final messages and wishes should be carefully recorded in a notebook designated for that purpose. So as soon as she could see Private Simpson beginning to slip away, Boon fetched the ward notebook and sat on a little stool by his bed, her head bent in close to hear, writing down as many of his last words and whispers as she could understand. Then, after he was gone, she found the chaplain and made sure she knew the location of his grave. Then she wrote to his mother.

Boon had arrived at the front in 1916, one of the new nursing intake brought over for the Somme offensive. Two years on and she had written so many sympathy letters that she had lost count. All she knew was that she had to make sure she didn't get behind with them. A colleague tried to write at least a dozen letters a night, but during the battle of Arras he had got behind and had to write almost sixty letters in one night to catch up.[24] Another nurse wrote almost 400 letters during Passchendaele, and a German-speaking nurse composed almost as many in the POW ward at her CCS. Battles and deaths in winter were the worst, when the freezing wind blew through their tents and gutted their candles. They had to warm the bottle of frozen ink in their hands or beg a pan of hot water from the kitchen before they could begin the work of writing.

Nurses had come to understand that their letters to the families of the deceased did not mark the end of their care. Families replied with questions and requests for further details. They asked what the weather had been like at the funeral, about what hymns had been sung, how many mourners had been there and what the chaplain had said. Boon had got used to the many questions that families asked about the last hours of her patients – what they had said, whether they had been in pain, where they were buried – and she tried to anticipate them in her letters. But it wasn't always possible to address all their concerns and sometimes her correspondence with the bereaved would continue for months.[25] If their loved ones were buried during heavy offensives, Boon had to make a little information go a long way. And she always hoped they wouldn't ask about coffins. No family liked to know about the brown blankets in which the dead were wrapped for burial. If they had an image in their head of their loved one being laid to rest in a sturdy coffin of French oak, Boon was happy for them to hold onto it.

Once she had finished the letter, she looked around the quiet ward. It was true when she wrote to the families that the patient's last hours were spent in warmth and comfort, made largely painless by drugs.[26] And, most of all, they weren't alone. Boon had come to understand quite soon after she arrived in France that nurses were always there at the end. Once a casualty had been given a note of DI or SI, he would receive no further visits from the doctor. Doctors had barely enough time for the men they could save. Those they couldn't were gently moved into the moribund ward and, from then on, it was the nurses who comforted and cared for them, along with the chaplain. Here death was their responsibility.

It was time for the ward round. But before she set out, Boon turned to the clipboard with the SI/DI patient list that hung outside the Sister's office. She entered the information for Private Simpson and scanned the list to see if any of the other patients might need morphine or if their condition was likely to worsen. The list was scrupulously maintained so that nurses changing shift and the chaplains could see at a glance who was likely to die on their watch. She put the ward notebook next to the list, so that other nurses could record the last murmurings of their patients. She nodded at the orderlies who came in as silently as they could to take Private Simpson away.

Then she quietly walked past each bed. There were many things she might be called upon to do for her patients. Often it was help with sipping a drink or some balm for cracked lips and drying skin. Some were so weak they couldn't brush the hair out of their eyes, so Boon always had a comb tucked in her pocket. Once a boy had cried out and she thought she must have missed his morphine dose, but when she got to his bed, he gasped that his lavender bag had fallen on the floor and he could suddenly smell his own decay. She picked up the bag and pinned it on the pillow next to his face. The boy immediately turned his head towards it and began to inhale the clean scent. He died a short while afterwards.

But tonight it was quiet. The dying men slept silently, with no raving or weeping, their shallow breaths occasionally catching before resuming. Boon returned to her desk and began the last job nurses ever did for their patients. In a laundry basket on the floor were the clean uniforms of the dead, and the linen bags that contained their personal possessions. She put each soldier's uniform and belongings into a bag, carefully pulled the drawstring and then labelled it for the mail office to send it home. Even if she had already written to the family, Boon always tried to put a final letter inside and looked in the ward notebook to remind herself of the dead man. Until her ward was empty, it was up to her to hold each ending in her memory, for as long as she could, so that the families would have more than a drawstring bag and a tattered tunic as the last remnants of their loved one.

7

Orderlies

Alfred Arnold, Harold Foakes

The glorious victories and advances of the last week have meant much work for the Royal Army Medical Corps.

Alfred Arnold, September 1916

Alfred Arnold was called up in the spring of 1916. As a school-teacher, and therefore regarded as capable of learning technical skills, he was offered the chance to train as an RAMC orderly. The Army needed hundreds more medical staff for the planned summer offensives, and Arnold needed a post that gave him the weekends off during training. He was the last of his farmer father's three sons to be conscripted and, once he stopped helping out on the land, there was no one else except his mother. When he finally got his orders for France in May, he told his mother not to worry: RAMC men were almost never put in danger and he would keep an eye on his two brothers already posted there. On a map he showed her that his casualty clearing station was likely to be miles from the action. She still cried without stopping as he boarded the train at Cambridge.

It took Arnold a while to travel through France, via the huge training camp at Étaples and changing trains at identically chaotic railheads, but when he found himself on the last leg of the journey he settled back and looked out of the window at the landscape passing by. He had expected everything about France to be different, but the land looked surprisingly like that at home. His father farmed Cambridgeshire fenland – flat as far as the eye could see – and here too there were flat fields, tall with early-summer crops, and dotted among them he could see men and women working. He even recognised what they were growing (rye mostly) and how long it would take until the crops were ready for harvesting, allowing for the differences in the weather between France and home. But as the train approached the front line, a major difference became obvious: the farmers at home didn't have to worry about gun emplacements and observation posts, which seemed to punch their way up through the soil like stone fists. But the French farmers evidently ignored them. Arnold could see rye planted right up to the edge of the concrete walls.

At the railhead Arnold was met by a lorry sent from the CCS. There were already nurses and other orderlies in the back, squeezed up on wooden benches, clutching kitbags or little suitcases. Like him, they were part of the preparations for the coming offensive. Hesitant introductions soon turned into chatter as they bumped along a muddy track. Notes were compared. Arnold impressed them all as he listed his skills, courtesy of the new RAMC training. Not only could he treat a range of battlefield injuries, but he was trained to give injections, assist the surgeons and provide basic anaesthetics.

Arnold's CCS consisted of long, neat rows of sturdy tents pitched near a river so that it had a readily available water supply. All around were the same flat fields of rye he had seen from the train, and the only landmark against the horizon was a concrete observation post, with a single track cut through the crop leading up to it. It was a familiar setting and made Arnold feel a little more comfortable. But it would be weeks before he got to use any of his medical training. They had discovered that the river was polluted with sewage, so holes for water tanks had to be dug, and water brought in lorries from a well at a farmhouse some distance away. Then there was the bumpy track leading to the CCS, which was barely passable for the little traffic that was using it so far; it would be completely useless for the large numbers of ambulances bringing casualties once the offensive had begun. When a unit of French soldiers arrived, Arnold was sent to work with them building a new road. They started at the main highway several miles away – Arnold saw how it was choked with gun crews and supply vehicles – and by the time they had finished there was a smooth, straight road leading directly into the heart of the CCS. Arnold's technical expertise had ensured that it was wide enough, with parking areas close to the taking-in tents, and that it connected with all the CCS's paths. It turned out to be an important job and Arnold was proud of his contribution.

But then, just as they finished, orders came for the CCS to move. A map and coordinates were enclosed and, when the officers sat down to work out their destination, it was found to be less than a mile away from where they were now, on the other side of the polluted river. But orders were orders, and they moved their tents and equipment. Arnold went out again with the road-builders and extended the road to their new site. Until June they moved several times to a new location never very far from their old one. It drove Arnold mad, but he learned how to pitch a tent in short order and he now knew every inch of canvas in the CCS. And however much they moved, he could still see the observation post somewhere in the distance. In June he noticed more and more soldiers winding their way through the track in the corn to the concrete tower, back and forth. It was clear that something was coming and it was close.

On the morning of 1 July the staff gathered outside and looked across the fields, towards the sound of the bombardment. They had begun their own preparations sometime before. They had squeezed as many stocks of dressings, drugs, bed linen and food as they could into the storage tents. Fresh graves were dug a discreet distance away, and all the stretchers and blankets that could be found were assembled outside the tents in case they soon filled up. They did one final round of the tented wards, looking at the rows of freshly made beds waiting to be filled. Then they waited. No casualties arrived on the first day of the offensive. Or on the second day. They waited for almost a week, feeling increasingly frustrated, constantly asking each other what they thought had happened because there was no one else to ask. The answer was horribly simple: the many thousands of wounded and dying men had so overwhelmed the casualty retrieval system that it took days before ambulances could begin properly distributing the patients to the CCSs.

Then, on 7 July, it all happened at once. From a never-ending stream of ambulances coming up the new road, 330 men were admitted in just one day. Suddenly Arnold was needed everywhere at once, running from the operating theatre to the receiving area and back again. He opened the back of one ambulance after another to supervise the unloading and taking-in of the wounded men. The delay in getting casualties to the CCSs meant that most of the vehicles were full of men who had dressings that were two or three days old, and who had eaten nothing but biscuits and the scrapings of old bully-beef tins for a week. One of the drivers warned him that when he opened the back of the ambulance the smell would make him reel backwards, let alone the sight of men torn apart. Arnold hadn't had time for breakfast and he was grateful for it.

From the ambulances, Arnold brought the casualties to one of the receiving tents, where he joined the other orderlies and nurses in removing the rags of uniforms and cleaning the wounded men. A doctor assessed each patient, and Arnold usually followed those who needed immediate surgery into the surgical tents. The operating theatre was running twenty-four hours a day. More often than not, a surgeon looked up as Arnold brought in a man on his trolley and told him they were short of surgical orderlies, or could he get the patient under. Arnold had to find enough water to wash himself and clean a set of anaesthetic equipment. Then, after surgery, it was back to the receiving tent. If he was lucky he got a bit of dinner over the next few days, a sandwich from the padre or a tin of stew, but often he went to bed hungry, with no certainty of having time for breakfast the next day.

The CCS had changed beyond recognition from the silence just a few days earlier. Now everything was noise. There was the crying and choking of the patients, staff calling out to each other, trying to find equipment, dressings or a spare pair of hands. Only one tent in the entire place was silent. It was where he and the other orderlies prepared the dead for their funerals. Inside there were three long tables and a pile of cloth bags, each containing a printed form. For each corpse Arnold took a bag and a form. He removed the dead man's uniform, if it was worth saving, and any possessions that he had in his pockets and placed them carefully in the bag. Then he filled out the form using the soldier's identity tags or tickets. If the uniform needed laundering before it was returned to the family, he stored it separately. Then he washed the body, smoothed down the hair, straightened out the stiffened limbs. Finally he took one of the neatly folded brown blanket coffins. With another orderly, he bundled the dead man in it, and together they took his body round to a cart waiting outside the tent and wheeled it to the cemetery.

Arnold hated the death tent. He hated the silence that bore down on him as soon as he stepped inside. He hated it more than opening the back of the worst-smelling ambulance, more than taking a barrowful of amputated limbs from theatre to the incinerator. As bad as all those things were, they were about living men. Death was gaining power over Arnold, and he tried to resist by growing himself a hard shell behind which to retreat. But he never quite managed it. Only the death tent made him cry. By the eighth day of the Somme offensive, most of the ambulances contained nothing but the dying and the dead. Arnold rarely went into the receiving tent now, but brought the men straight to the awful silence of the death tent. There he and the other orderlies worked, all day and late into the night, the silence interrupted only by the faint sound of their crying as they loaded watches, diaries and photographs into the simple cloth bags marked with the names of the dead.

It took a fortnight to clear the first batch of patients, with staff sleeping when they could on legged stretchers that kept them up off the wet grass. When the last patient had gone, they heard that another wave was on its way, so the whole station had to be cleaned. Arnold shared the mopping and scrubbing work with the most senior surgeons and MOs, down on their knees, muddying their theatre scrubs. No one spoke of the blood that stained the water in their buckets for sweep after sweep.

Supplies were low and Arnold was sent to find more. Go towards the front, someone said, there's plenty of stuff lying around where it was dumped, where they couldn't find anyone to deliver it to. He took a lorry and soon found several abandoned supply dumps full of food and water. When he got out of the cab to load them up, he stopped in his tracks as the battlefield spread out before him. He didn't know how long he stood there on an otherwise beautiful summer's day, staring at the dead, the wire, the fields blown to pieces. Surely no one could ever sow or plough again on that land. Then there was the smell. The whole place reeked of decomposition, as if there was not enough wind in the world to blow it all away.[1] Arnold pulled himself together and loaded up the lorry. He made several other stops whenever he saw anything that looked useful but tried not to let his eyes wander across the landscape and focused on the road, instead. A railhead was his last stop and there he thought he saw the worst sight of all. An ordinary train, similar to the one that had brought him to the front, was at one end unloading reinforcements, while at the other end it was filling up with wounded men.

Back at the CCS, the next 300 casualties that had arrived were in far worse condition than the first lot. Almost all of them died before making it even to the moribund ward, so day after day Arnold was either at the cemetery with the padre or working in the death tent, sorting through possessions, labelling them for home and crying silently. There were so many sets of belongings to be sorted that they had to ask the bearers to help them. They tried not to cry in front of them when they saw their rough hands filling a bag with ID tags, pay books and all the personal things that would have meant so much to the dead soldier. Arnold had great respect for the bearers. They saw so much more death than he did, and still they would help him in the death tent. Then they would help the padre with the funerals, filling in the graves and paying their respects at the short ceremony.

One afternoon he went for a walk in the fields when suddenly he realised that it was August. Harvest had already begun here, earlier than at home. He stood on the edge of a rye field and reached out to feel the grain in the palm of his hand. It was extraordinary how the French farmers harvested with the noise of the guns in the background. If he concentrated on them swishing slowly against the rye with their scythes, perhaps he could forget the war, too. He watched a farmer putting a sheaf on a pile. It wasn't sheaved as neatly as it was at home, he noticed, so it wouldn't be as easy to stack. Then he looked beyond the field to the road and he could see another line of ambulances driving towards the CCS. He needed to go back.

A third 'great push' at the Somme filled the hospital with more casualties and Arnold soon forgot about the fields and the harvest. He didn't forget about home, though, and sometimes the hope of a parcel or letter with a Cambridge postmark waiting on his bed in his tent was the only thing that kept him going. They had all been ordered not to keep letters, and accordingly he burned them – but only after reading them so many times that the paper was almost worn through. His family also sent provisions. His mother's home-made cake, gingerbread, biscuits and chocolate all found their way from the Fens to the French rye fields in time for his birthday in September. One morning a little square cardboard box arrived, containing a slice of fruit cake from the wedding of a childhood friend. He sat alone in his tent and ate it to the last crumb, toasting the couple as he went.

In September the casualties continued to come thick and fast. It was still hot and the heat and the blood brought swarms of flies. It felt worse than being in a butcher's shop. For one whole week the heavy guns pounded day and night, far closer than ever before, adding terror and exhaustion to the woes afflicting the CCS staff. One day a film crew pitched up and filmed a couple of scenes for a film they were making about the battle of the Somme. Arnold thought it was ridiculous – surely no one would pay to see the kind of work he did every day.

On Sundays they got their cigarette ration and a delivery of fresh fruit. If there was time, Arnold would go to one of the padre's services – one that wasn't a funeral – and he felt that those moments of worship in the fields sustained him remarkably. The farm, the family and the church had been the cornerstones of his life in Cambridgeshire and, in a strange sort of way, they remained so in France. His parents did their best to support him. They kept up with all his requests: for pen nibs, underwear, mousetraps, brilliantine for his hair, and sausages to cook on a little grill that had been rigged up in his tent. They sent so many parcels that he asked for the postage to be paid out of his wages, which his family were looking after, but they never did. In return he did his best to keep them up to date with the progress of his brothers at the front. One had been wounded at Thiepval, so Arnold tracked him down and visited him at the CCS. His brother's wound wasn't severe, he was happy to report, and he went back to his unit after a couple of weeks.

October brought lighter loads, and the weather changed almost overnight. With the cold and rain came requests home from Arnold for warm clothes and underwear. The little grill in the tent worked tirelessly, producing toast, cocoa and sausages for the grateful staff who gathered around it, once the theatres were closed and the patients asleep. Such moments lifted Arnold's spirits. Above all, happiness had the power to astound him more than any of the human misery he witnessed on a daily basis. He felt it when he was sitting down with his colleagues, joking about the day, pouring out cocoa. And when he walked through a town amongst local people going about their business, with not a single soldier in sight, he was surprised to feel peaceful and relaxed. The world still turned, and he realised he was still capable of happiness. Such small miracles almost took his breath away.

By November the number of casualties arriving at the CCS was getting smaller and smaller. There was more of what Arnold called 'soft time', with few or no patients and nothing much to do. Yet they had become so accustomed to the heavy loads, to the pressure and the desire to save lives, that without the endless stream of casualties, the CCS seemed to lack purpose. Some staff hoped the lull meant that the war would be over soon. But Arnold thought differently: the war had become routine and a dull one at that, despite all the suffering.

When there was an outbreak of flu, every single member of staff was struck down, one after the other, the rows of beds filling with nurses and orderlies, not soldiers. All of them worried what would happen if another load of casualties suddenly arrived. Thankfully, no ambulances pulled up. By now Arnold was growing bored with the routine of soft time. He got up at six-thirty, had breakfast and then spent most of the day endlessly cleaning the surgical tent and all the instruments. He checked supplies and followed the doctors and surgeons on their ward round. He didn't like a full operating theatre, but he liked an empty one even less. He felt his training was going to waste and started to think that he ought to be closer to the action.

When Arnold learned that the Somme offensive had finally come to a halt in November, he made up his mind. It didn't look as if there would be much more for him to do at the CCS, so he asked for a posting to a field ambulance, where he could follow the war and its wounded more closely. When the transfer came through, he burned the last of his letters from home and passed on the little grill that had sustained them all, together with instructions not to burn the tent down and to boil the sausages before grilling them, for safety's sake. He caught a lift from an ambulance going to the railhead and, as they drove away, his eyes once more turned to the fields around them, full of grey stubble after the harvest, the concrete emplacements still stark and hard against the darkened winter sky. In other fields women dug potatoes, their backs breaking with the work, their men all somewhere in the trenches. When he finally arrived at the front, he found it as he remembered it from his supply runs: the land smashed and barren – a very different harvest scythed down across the valley. Arnold stayed with the field ambulance until the end of the war, working on patients who were alive. He never minded the noise of the battle or the chaos of constant movement. Anything was better than the silence of death.

Easter of 1917 brought heavy snow and freezing temperatures as the Arras offensive ground to a halt over a bloody pile of 20,000 casualties.[2] Medical teams were at full stretch, working day and night. Lance Corporal Harold Foakes had been posted as battalion orderly to the 13th Royal Fusiliers stationed outside Monchy-le-Preux. He worked closely with the battalion's MOs, trying to keep up with the influx of casualties, rolling bandages and checking on supplies. By Easter Monday there were only Foakes, one MO and some bearers left working at the dressing station. Then the devastating news came that their last six stretcher bearers had been killed on a carry by a single shell. Yet the desperate cries of wounded men stuck out on the battlefield continued. Foakes watched as the MO put the strap of one heavy medical pannier over his shoulder and then lifted up a second. He wondered how the man would manage with the two panniers weighing him down like that, as he set out across the mangled ground, in the snow and ice, towards the cries that came through the freezing air.

Foakes was now the only medically skilled man left working at the station, and as the hours went by he realised that the doctor wasn't coming back. But the wounded were still calling out, in sobs of pain and terror, and someone had to try to reach them. He waited a little while longer, hoping help would materialise from somewhere. When it didn't, he looked at his supplies. There were three panniers, full of dressings, iodine, bandages, water and morphine; he would try and carry them all. He would also need food for men stuck without supplies. No rations had been delivered for a while, but there were some biscuits that he'd been saving and a jar of jam. He stuffed it all down inside one of the panniers and buckled it up tight. There was a folded tarpaulin in the corner of the station, so he'd take that, too. It didn't weigh much and you never knew when it could be useful. He took a deep breath as he stood up straight under the weight of his burdens. Then he headed out of the tent.

Outside in the snow some soldiers were waiting for him. They had gone over the top that day and made it back, but they all knew someone who hadn't, who might still be lying in a shell hole, calling out. Foakes saw big men, grimy-faced, nodding encouragement. There were snipers on the other side, they told him, but they would cover him until he was safe. He had to make it to the boys out there: they depended on him. The soldiers even called him 'Doc', giving him a kind of battlefield promotion. As Foakes climbed the ladder out onto the field, men with rifles on either side of him guarded him as far as they could. There was some gunfire, but he made it to one of the shell holes, rolling down and crouching at the bottom. Now he was alone, with no one to protect him.

Foakes unloaded his panniers and rubbed his aching shoulders. No one had been shooting directly at him, so he reckoned it was safe enough to put up the little red-cross pennant that he found in one of the panniers to show where he was. He tied it to a stick and, crawling up to the rim of the hole, planted it as firmly as he could in some soft mud. The little pennant immediately began cracking and fluttering in the wind, but didn't attract any fire. Foakes raised his head to get his bearings. He could no longer see the trenches he had come from, or the dressing station. It was as if he had entered another world. The ground was white and brown, snow and mud all around, with more snow falling all the while. He squinted to see more precisely what was around him and thought he could make out an arm waving at him in the distance. There were cries of 'Over here, Doc, we're over here'. Then, suddenly, shots rang out, cracking sharply close by. He wriggled back down to safety at the bottom of the hole and thought about what to do next.

Foakes began by turning the shell hole into a medical post. He unpacked the panniers and dug into the frosted earth to store the dressings, bandages and medications. He knelt upright and looked at his work: it would have to do. Now for the casualties. He slowly climbed to the edge of the shell hole and crawled out. He kept as low as possible, moving in the direction of the last cry he had heard. Whoever had been shooting at him didn't see him, so he kept going. The cry had come from a shell hole, but when he rolled over its rim and landed in the mud, he almost cried out in despair. There wasn't just one but nine men at the bottom, each badly wounded and some close to death. Foakes gathered himself and stayed with them for a moment, trying to reassure them and leaving behind his water canteen. Then he crawled back to his improvised medical post. None of the men were able to move, so he would have to carry them somehow.

He remembered the tarpaulin he had brought: he would turn it into a stretcher. He crawled out of his post again and, on his journey across the battlefield, it occurred to him that if you worry about snipers you don't have time to worry about getting wet, cold or muddy. When he returned to the wounded soldiers, Foakes took the first man who called out to him and rolled him in the tarpaulin, tying it round him with a piece of cord. Holding the end of the cord between his teeth and pulling the load over his shoulder, he set out across the battlefield towards his medical post, crawling and dragging the man behind him, and keeping himself as flat as he possibly could.

Five more times he went back and forth. With more snow falling, snipers firing and men crying in pain, each haul was taking an age. The tarpaulin became sodden with freezing water and stained with blood, and his body ached as five more times he braced himself for the weight of the wounded man and clenched the cord in his agonised jaw. When he returned for the seventh time the three remaining men were those most badly injured and least likely to survive the drag across the battlefield. There was nothing he could do for them except speak to them calmly, softly, brushing their hair out of their eyes and giving them a last injection of morphine. Then he waited until each had gone to a better place. He folded up the tarpaulin and returned for the final time to his medical post. It required no real effort this time, yet it felt like the hardest passage of all. When he got back to his shell hole, he got on with distributing supplies and cutting up dressings. No one asked him what had happened to the three men left behind.

It was two days before a stretcher bearer made it out to Foakes's post to offer his help and tell him that an MO was on his way and the battle had moved on. He found a functioning medical post, the tarpaulin now providing a roof against the snow and the men well cared for, waiting patiently to make the final leg of their journey. Foakes had made a fine medical officer, working almost without sleep, catching only a few minutes here and there. He told the bearer that he was fine, just a bit hungry with only his biscuits and jam to live off for three days. He had rationed them as carefully as his supplies of water and morphine. Carefully Foakes and the bearer started to pack up the post, ready to move it when the doctor arrived.

The doctor had got lost in the snow, but then he had seen Foakes's red-cross pennant, still fluttering in the icy winds of Arras. With the doctor came bearer teams, and eventually everyone got back to the medical post behind the lines where an ambulance was waiting to move the casualties on. Foakes's stint as a doctor was over, but he didn't mind returning to his orderly duties. When he looked back out over the battlefield he wondered how he had ever survived, let alone kept six men alive for three days. Then the MO called to him and he went back inside the tent to dress more wounds.

8

Wounded

John Glubb, Menin Road, 21 August 1917

The real horrors of war were to be seen in the hospitals, not on the battlefield.

John Glubb, August 1917

As the third battle of Ypres lurched into its third week, another Allied offensive shambled to a bloody halt. Orders were sent round to all officers that because of the proximity of enemy guns, they were not to ride horses close to the front. Too many officers had already been lost and those that remained shouldn't turn themselves into easy targets. John Glubb, a young lieutenant in the Royal Engineers, ignored the orders. He loved being on horseback. He could cut through the traffic jams that built up behind the lines and find gaps through which supplies could move forward.[1] He also thought it was important for him to be seen at the front, without fear, as it gave the men confidence – something in short supply in the third week of August 1917 at Passchendaele. So for almost a week Glubb rode on, day and night, supervising the repair of roads and moving supplies up to the line. He didn't particularly like his horse, a young mare called Geisha, which shied and whinnied at every little thing, but he was needed everywhere at once and being on horseback was by far the most efficient means of getting around.

On 21 August he was sent to look for a wagonload of equipment that was supposed to be somewhere on the congested

Hénin–Saint-Martin-sur-Cojeul road. He had pulled up briefly to lean in through a cab window to ask a lorry driver if he had seen the supplies when a shell exploded nearby, lifting him off Geisha's back and tossing him high in the air. He later remembered landing slowly back on his horse, before tumbling to the ground. Then he got angry because it felt as if someone had punched him or hit him across the face with a cricket bat. It must have been that bloody horse he never liked, he thought, which had kicked him and cut his face with her shoe.

But it wasn't Geisha (who was terrified but uninjured, and had galloped for safety as soon as Glubb let go of her reins). Instead he had been injured by the fragments of the shell that had exploded just ahead of him, its metal debris hitting his mouth and neck. He struggled to his feet, trying to pull himself together. He waited for a while to see what would happen next. He realised he had been deafened, but when he managed to stay on his feet he decided to head for the crossroads where, despite all the chaos, he remembered he had seen a medical post in an old cellar. He should be able to get there, he thought. He was surprised that he wasn't feeling any pain, although there was the weird sound of swishing liquid pumping rhythmically close to his ear: at least his hearing was beginning to return. When he lifted his hand he saw there was blood running down his sleeve, dripping off his fingers.[2]

The lorry driver to whom Glubb had been talking came running over to the crumpled heap lying in a pool of blood. Another driver came to help, taking Glubb's arm and putting it over his shoulders, trying not to look at his smashed face. Glubb stuttered some words, but the man didn't understand. The driver also remembered the medical post in the cellar and together they brought the young officer there.

There was no MO at the dressing station, just an orderly. But three weeks at Passchendaele had provided him with his own medical qualification, so he was perfectly capable of running the post himself. He took Glubb from the lorry driver and helped him lie down on the battered pine table in the middle of the dressing station. He gently turned his head from side to side. He had seen some sights that day, but this face was one of the very worst. The left side of the jaw was all but gone, torn away by the shrapnel from the shell, and there were bits of bone and teeth strewn in the wreckage. Everything below the nose was torn from its moorings, including an artery, from which was pumping fresh red blood just below the ear: this was the swishing sound that Glubb had heard when he was kneeling in the road. At least it told the orderly where to start. Same priority as always: stop the bleeding. He carefully put a bandage in place to plug the torn artery. Glubb could no longer hear the swishing sound of his life draining away. Then the orderly dressed the wound as best he could, covering the debris, holding it in place.

He knew there was nothing more he could do. Glubb had to be taken to a casualty clearing station as soon as possible, but there was no ambulance. Walking was the only option, but the wounded man would never make it on his own. So the orderly made a swift decision: he would close the dressing station and take Glubb to the CCS himself. He helped Glubb off the table and they set off, the younger man leaning on the orderly's arm, barely capable of registering each step. Along the way they stumbled across another medical dugout. The MO there only needed to look at Glubb to know that he wouldn't be able to walk much further. The orderly must find an ambulance or Glubb would die; it was a miracle that he was still alive. As luck would have it, there was an ambulance ready to leave for the nearest CCS. The loss of blood was starting to tell and Glubb began to feel cold. What remained of his teeth began to chatter. He still wasn't in any pain, but feeling his broken jaw and floating teeth was strange and deeply unpleasant. He grunted and pointed at the MO's notepad. Writing shakily, he asked the MO to let his unit know that he was injured. The MO nodded. When the ambulance pulled away with Glubb in the back, heading for No. 20 CCS at Ficheux, he sent a wire to his battalion saying that Glubb was badly wounded and probably wouldn't last the day.

But he did last. Thanks to the experienced nurses at No. 20, he lived as long as the next morning, and then long enough to be wheeled into theatre for surgery. Glubb remembered orderlies carrying his stretcher along the muddy paths, and seeing the blue sky and drifting white clouds above him. It would be his last pleasant memory for quite some time. It was always difficult to anaesthetise a facial casualty, and when they used a huge rubber mask to flood his face with ether they had to guess at the right amounts. On the table Glubb began to hallucinate and felt that he was being suffocated. The surgery itself would be even worse. The repair of his jaw was much more difficult than the surgeon had anticipated and Glubb kept stirring awake and needed to be re-anaesthetised. Because of all the movement on the operating table, his tongue kept flopping about, getting in the way of the surgeon's instruments, so he pinned a rod through it to keep it still. When Glubb came to after the operation he couldn't believe that the pain was worse than when he went into surgery – and now his tongue was swollen as well. He could hardly breathe, was unable to talk and no longer understood what was happening to him.

When the orderly returned him to his bed in the ward Glubb tried to calm his mind. It was almost impossible. Everything the nurses usually did to make things more comfortable for their patients made his life more intolerable. A gramophone had been set up in the tent, playing jolly tunes all day long. But to Glubb it sounded like incessant tinny scratchings, like an insect stuck in his ear that would not be dislodged. His senses had suddenly been tuned to an excruciating level. Every touch – however kind or gentle – became a burn, every sound a screech. To make things worse, the man in the bed next to him had been injured in the head and screamed gibberish for hours on end.[3] Glubb would easily have throttled him, if he had had the strength to get out of bed. His wound kept bleeding, but the nurses were too busy for regular dressing changes, leaving him lying in his own discharge, with its rank smell.

After a couple of days he finally managed to make himself understood through the bandages and gradually his senses returned to their normal state. It helped that he had plenty of visitors. His father, who was stationed nearby, came often, as did his comrades and his CO. His batman took away the clothes he had been wearing when he was hit and did his best to get the bloodstains out so that he would have something to wear for the journey home. Then, almost a week after he had been wounded, orderlies collected him for transportation to the hospital train. But nobody changed his dressings before he left, so he began the next phase of his journey with a set that were already twenty-four hours old.

From then on, Glubb's journey got worse and worse. It was too complicated to feed him in transit, but he was lying in the train carriage next to the kitchen and could smell food all day and all night. He had never known hunger like it. He wanted to shout at the nurses who walked past him, carrying trays of food, to stop torturing him. The liquids they gave him by dropper were no consolation and nothing like enough. After twelve hours his dressing turned septic, but he was the only one who noticed. The smell of his own infected tissue made him want to weep.[4] He tried to call out, but the noise of the train and the cries of the other patients drowned him out. Because he wasn't on the meal roster, no one stopped by his bunk on a regular basis, and so there he lay, starving and ignored.

The hospital ship that bore him to England wasn't much better. It was desperately understaffed, and rather than remove and entirely re-dress his wounds, a distracted nurse just added another layer of bandages. By the time they docked at Southampton he had an enormous white turban wrapped round his head. He looked like no other casualty on the boat, and a crowd gathered to watch as he was unloaded. When he was left on the dock for a while, surrounded by a silent crowd of spectators, Glubb could see the blue sky overhead, but at least this time it was English sky. Then there was no room on the hospital trains that ran directly between the coast and the London mainline stations, so he was berthed in a window seat in an ambulance carriage hitched up behind an ordinary passenger train, stopping at all its regular stations. At every single stop his turban drew a crowd. He couldn't move away from the window and the attention, so he closed his eyes and tried to sleep.

He woke to find himself on a stretcher at Victoria Station, looking up to see the huge iron roof above him, its cavern filled with shouting and steam. Then the face of a nurse in a dark-blue cape appeared overhead. She explained that she was from the London Ambulance Column and would be taking him to the 3rd London General Hospital in Wandsworth. He did his best to nod under his turban. It was a beautiful evening, and she would leave the back doors of the ambulance open, so that he could see the late-September sun and all the people waiting to greet him. When the ambulance turned out of the shade of the station into the evening's light, suddenly there was cheering all around them. Lifting his head, he saw crowds of men and women lining the streets, waving when they saw him, calling out that he was brave and they were proud of him. Tweed caps were waved, flowers were thrown and there was singing. Wave after wave of applause followed each little ambulance leaving the station. The nurse could only see his eyes but she could tell that, for the first time in a long while, pain had been replaced by pride and hope.[5]

9

Chaplains

Wilfred Abbott, Ernest Crosse, Charles Doudney, John Murray, Cyril Horsley-Smith, Montagu Bere, John Lane Fox

If a chaplain arrives at a bearer post, offer him a job to do. In addition to his own duties, he will be glad to give assistance and usually does it well.

Letter from 'Captain', *Journal of the Royal Army Medical Corps*, 1916[1]

After Neuve Chapelle, when the doctor in the battered farmhouse remembered the days of blood and slaughter, one thing stayed most vividly in his mind. On the third day, a Sunday, he had begun to believe that the trail of broken men on stretchers would never end. Then something else. A bicycle bumped to a halt in the courtyard, carrying a tall, thin man, in uniform. As he dismounted, he took a moment to look around and smiled, a flash of sunlight suddenly glinting off his spectacles. He found an intact wall and carefully leaned the bicycle up against it, checking that it would balance, all the while ignoring the shells flying overhead. No one watching could quite see why he was taking so much trouble. Some of the onlookers recognised the bicycle, which looked as battered as the farmhouse, and the man. It was Wilfred Abbott, chaplain to the Gordons. They had seen him the day before when he had waved to them while cycling towards the front line to help the few remaining bearer teams remove the wounded. Then a huge shell had thumped into the ground close by. The soldiers rushed over, expecting only to find his mortal remains, but Abbott was somehow intact, with not even a scratch on his glasses. He dusted off his uniform and got back on his battered bicycle. Ignoring their pleas to return to the rear, he cycled off into the shelling as if he were out for a constitutional in a peaceful English lane. Now he was back again, still not blown to pieces.

The padre asked the doctor if he could help, but the medic's mind was too full with the noise and chaos of the aid post to be able to think of anything. What about a prayer? asked Abbott. The doctor noticed that things had suddenly grown quiet around him. The guns had found another target for the moment and the casualties seemed a little calmer. He nodded. Abbott went back to his bicycle and returned with some hymn sheets, and the doctor gathered everyone round. It would be a mixed congregation, he thought, not large, but definitely in need. Mostly it was medics and orderlies, their aprons and uniforms caked in mud and worse, with blood on their hands, arms and faces where they had tried to wipe away sweat and dust. A few casualties had also shuffled forward and held out their bandaged hands for the hymn sheets. Bearers sat down on the ground beside the men on stretchers to share the pages. They watched closely as Abbott pitched the first note and then they sang, weakly at first, but slowly becoming more confident. The guns started again, but the small congregation finished the hymn.

Then Abbott preached, for just long enough, about how God had given them an opportunity to do something useful. That their lives were no longer trivial, but important and they should give thanks for such a gift. The padre's eyes grew brighter as he drew the congregation towards him, and for a few moments his listeners felt that they were lifted away from the farmhouse and the battle. Then a few seconds of silence and the final Amen. The doctor was grateful to the strange, brave man with spectacles and the small, neat marks of his calling stitched on his uniform. When he went forward to shake the padre's hand, he found that a line of men had formed behind him to do the same. Then Abbott climbed back on his bicycle and rode on, in search of others who might need him.

In his short sermon on the last day of Neuve Chapelle, Abbott had expressed his own thanks for the gift of service that he had been given. An army chaplain's post hadn't seemed like much of a gift when he arrived in France in September 1914. He had received no training and there wasn't even anyone to meet him when he arrived in camp. It was the same for every chaplain who arrived in France in those first few days of the war. Some just retreated to their tents to wait for Sunday. But for Abbott and others waiting was not enough, so they looked for something to do. After all, they had come here to serve. They found that the only people who were actually pleased to see them were the Regimental Medical Officers – and they gave the chaplains something to do straight away.[2] It was with the RMOs, in the front line or to the rear, that Abbott and other padres found meaningful work and a new and extraordinary opportunity of service.[3]

Chaplain Ernest Crosse considered himself lucky, getting a front-line posting from the outset with the 7th/8th Battalion of the Devonshires. And he got what he most wanted: the opportunity to work with the battalion doc and make himself useful. For his part, the doctor was delighted to have a competent and professional man at his side – and Crosse never said no to anything. He tagged along with the bearers, an extra pair of hands and a strong back to bring in a casualty. Sometimes he walked in front, directing them away from broken duckboards and shell holes. He was particularly useful at night, when he took charge of the torch and its batteries and found them a path in the pitch dark. When he wasn't helping them with their carry, he was out on the battlefield, trying to get to know their sector. He scouted out new routes from the front to their aid post and made notes of any trenches that needed repairing. He also got himself a whistle so that he could alert the bearers if he came across a casualty that he couldn't bring in himself.

Crosse wasn't the only padre who made himself useful with the bearer teams. Chaplains had enough organisational skills and authority to round up volunteers either from the troops or, as they often spoke German, from newly captured POWs. They became so expert at organising and helping bearers that, if there was no medical officer available, padres were often given overall command of the battalion's bearer teams.[4] One chaplain, who would later win a VC for his service with bearers at the Somme, created an entire team from scratch after all the original members had been killed. When they got stuck in shell holes trying to retrieve the wounded, he ran back between them and the line to bring up supplies, seemingly ignoring the incessant, murderous shellfire. On one occasion the bearers saw him creeping towards them in an odd crouched posture. At first they thought he might be wounded, but then they realised that he was carrying a canteen of hot tea for the group, covering its top with one hand to protect it from flying mud.[5]

Once word arrived of the planned July offensive in the valley of the Somme, Crosse and the Devonshires' MO began to prepare medical posts and bearer routes. Then, on 30 June, they travelled together to the front-line trenches to make the final allocations of bearer teams. Crosse got back late that night and had only just fallen asleep when the barrage rang out signalling the advance. He jumped up and ran out of the dugout to say a few prayers with the men while they waited for the shriek of the whistle. It was to be the only religious duty he did all day. When the whistles blew and the men went over the top, Crosse made his way to the aid post, readying himself for the return of the wounded.

Right from the start the padre and the doc could see that things weren't going to plan. Worst of all, their aid post seemed to be in the wrong place. No casualties arrived all morning and they paced outside in frustration, waiting for bearers who didn't come. When the battalion commander passed by, they asked if they could go out onto the battlefield to look for casualties. They were strictly forbidden to do so. Far too many medics had already been killed out there. But as soon as the officer was out of sight they went anyway. When they made it to the first shell hole, ducking the whole way to avoid shellfire, they found four wounded men sheltering there. As the MO started to treat their injuries, Crosse called out across the line for bearers to come and help carry them back.

By the afternoon they decided to move their aid post closer to the men who needed them. They set out on a road that led them forward, closer to the battle line, but soon stopped in their tracks. The road before them was littered with bodies – injured men who had almost made it to safety, but died from their wounds. Before long the road took them onto the battlefield itself and they stopped again. From every shell hole they could see, right across the valley, there were men waving and they heard the cries of the wounded trapped there. They realised there were too many casualties to bring back on their own, so Crosse went looking for bearers. Back along the road he found leaderless teams who didn't know where to start, so he organised them into groups and showed them a meeting point to aim for when they returned with their carries. When they told him they didn't have enough stretchers, he got them to use the many trench ladders that had been abandoned after the troops had gone over the top. The padre made his way back to the doctor with thirty bearers. When he stumbled across an abandoned German dugout, he decided that it would be their new medical post. They took up residence, ready at last for the wounded.

The next day was very much the same. Doc and padre again searched the battlefield for casualties, and still every shell hole had broken men at the bottom. By now, all recognisable landmarks had been blasted away by the shelling, and Crosse had to make sure that he and the bearers didn't lose sight of each other and that they found their way back to the aid post. He could still see hands waving at them in the distance, men they wouldn't be able to reach. He tried to focus on those they could save.

On the afternoon of the third day Crosse left the battlefield and went to the new cemetery at Mansell Copse, where the dead of the Devonshires were to be buried. There 163 men were waiting for him, laid out in rows. He made sure that a sign was painted naming the place as the battalion cemetery. Then he inspected every single man to make sure that his identity tag and personal belongings had been properly stored. The bearers were still busy digging the last of the graves and Crosse checked that there would be a place for everyone, before returning to his dugout.

The following day he buried them all. The service took longer than expected as the guns continued to thunder around them and Crosse had to shout to make his words heard. He was told that the offensive had been successful, so he ended with a prayer of thanksgiving for the victory, but the sound of the guns made him doubt his own words. After the small congregation of comrades and officers had drifted away, Crosse took off his robes and joined the doctor and the bearers in filling in the graves. It took the rest of the day and they barely had the strength to make it back to their dugouts. Just before he fell asleep, Crosse looked at his hands. He had bearer hands now: worn, callused and so deeply stained with mud that he might never be able to get them clean. Worthy hands to hold a Bible and make the sign of the Cross, he thought.

Then the fighting began again, and this time it was even worse. Holding the north-east corner of the line, the Devonshires joined the battle for Delville Wood, and Crosse was ordered to lead bearer parties following the advance. Four of their number were soon killed and the terrain of torn woodland and churned ground brought their progress to a halt. When there was a lull in the fighting on 15 July, Crosse organised a sweep of the battlefield, stringing the bearers out in a long line. It was hard going, even though the guns had stopped, and mostly they found only corpses. By now there were no more mourners at Crosse's funerals, and no more prayers of thanksgiving.

On 21 July 1916 the Devonshires were finally relieved. Their journey had taken them from the Wellington Redoubt, through Mametz into Caterpillar Wood, Guillemont and finally to Delville

Wood. As the battalion headed to the rear, Crosse reflected on his work. Perhaps he should have concentrated more on his religious duties. Like many other padres at the front, weeks had gone by without services, only hurried prayers and funerals. One chaplain who moved up and down the line with a field ambulance did no religious work at all for several months. All his time was taken up looking after the walking wounded and, whenever they stopped to set up an aid post, it was his responsibility to oversee the unloading of the wagons and find supplies.[6] No one even thought to ask him if he wanted to conduct a service.

Instead there was often spontaneous religious activity. Crosse had heard of a medical officer who, having worked for days without stopping during the Somme, suddenly asked the battalion's chaplain for a Communion service. Their medical post had been set up in a requisitioned farm, so the padre held the service in a stable, some distance away from the dressing rooms full of bloody bandages and wounded men. Bales of hay insulated the tiny congregation briefly from the sounds of war, and the service was witnessed by the curious farm animals. Another padre had improvised a service for the six bearers in his team, reading from the Gospel of John about how every man's way in the world was lit by the coming of Christ, even if they were trudging through a bloody slough and death dogged their every step. Then they said a short prayer and went back to work.[7] The team had grown to like the padre, particularly when they came to understand that he wasn't there to preach at them. If the guns were especially threatening during a carry, he led them in singing hymns, loudly and in defiance, the rhythm helping them to keep pace as they marched.[8]

So when Crosse spent his first night for weeks on a clean, dry bed, he found that he had done his duty by his men, even if it wasn't quite what the Army Chaplains College had taught him. The next day he remembered that he had one more task to perform for the men of the Devonshires. He found an officer and begged his map of the Somme from him. Then he found a table and chair and spent his first morning away from the battle with the map spread out before him. He dug a nub of pencil out of his pocket and carefully marked down the location of the cemeteries and the graves of every man he had buried. When he had finished he gave the map to the CO. It was precious, he told him, and he should take good care not to lose it.

Charles Doudney didn't get a front-line posting, but he was happy to go wherever he might be useful. In fact, he had the potential to be very useful. He had been ordained at the age of twenty-three and immediately put in for missionary work. When he got a posting in the Australian Outback he was told that he needed some sound medical knowledge, because if the doctor wasn't available to his parishioners, then the vicar would have to step in. Doudney attached himself to the medical school of one of London's teaching hospitals for a term and walked the wards alongside the students. Thus properly prepared, he left for Australia, where for ten years he ministered to men and women who hacked out a living in the burning desert – and who indeed came to him when the doctor wasn't around.

His experience in the Outback taught him a great deal. He realised that he wasn't fazed by much and could gain the trust of hard-working men and women of few words. He also discovered that he was still good at science, which he had loved at school. His only means of communication in Australia had been an old radio set, which he was constantly mending and improving. When he returned to England he missed it so much that he built a new radio for himself, running the aerial up the steeple of his parish church in Bath to achieve a stronger signal. Over the next few years he became an expert in telegraphy and radio electronics, and when war broke out in August 1914 he passed on to the War Office the German signals traffic that he was picking up. It was no surprise to his parishioners when he announced from his pulpit that he would soon be off to serve with the British Expeditionary Force.

He arrived in France in early May 1915 and was first assigned to one of the base hospitals in Rouen.[9] There was no time for him to think how he would serve: that decision had already been made for him. The Artois offensive had begun and the hospital needed all the spare hands it could get. Doudney assumed he would be helping to unload ambulances, but word had got out that the new padre had an interest in radiology and a small tool kit in his luggage, containing a voltammeter, an ammeter and a soldering iron. Within days of his arrival at Rouen he had become chief repair man in the X-ray department, and as the hospital filled with patients he was soon given scrubs to put on over his army tunic and was made relief radiologist. Working alongside a surgeon, Doudney operated the equipment and offered his opinion on whether or not something caught on film was a shrapnel fragment. By the time the offensive came to an end he had worked on more than 100 patients and thousands of wounds. Even after the casualties had been moved on, he continued to spend a good part of every day in radiology, either with patients or repairing and testing equipment with his soldering iron and meters.

His skill and cool had made a considerable impression on the medical staff of the hospital and by the end of May Doudney was asked if he would help out with administering anaesthetics. He would of course be given the necessary training. Doudney agreed immediately: he didn't want this work to take up the valuable time of one of the doctors. There was no doubt in his mind that this was what he should be doing, even though he spent little time on his religious duties. But then he had never cared much about the details of ritual.[10] God was everywhere in the hospital: not just in the chapel, but in the radiology lab, the operating theatre and the wards. Writing home to his family, he told them that he found 'more than traces of God himself the Sufferer and the Healer in rough soldier and cultured doctor'. It was just as important for him to work in the medical wards, theatres and laboratories as it was to be holding services and taking Communion round. It was all God's work.[11] And Doudney wasn't the only chaplain asked to help with the wounded as part of his ministry. Many padres joined the bearers and attended the RMOs' weekly lectures to gain some medical knowledge. By the end of 1915 many chaplains knew a bearer's pannier as well as their prayer book, and soon wounded soldiers were no longer surprised when they saw that the man bending over them was a padre and not a doctor.[12]

In the summer of 1915 Doudney was posted to one of the new casualty clearing stations based in an old hop-store in Vlamertinghe near Poperinghe. Although it had the latest X-ray facilities and bacteriological labs, the CCS was short-staffed, with only three surgeons and six orderlies. All their MOs manned the aid posts at the front during the second phase of the Artois offensive. So once again Doudney's experience was desperately needed and he rolled up his sleeves and got to work. It was the first time since returning from Australia that he had been asked to treat patients without supervision and he was worried that he wasn't properly prepared. But there were many simple wounds that anyone could treat and he found that his medical training soon resurfaced.

Doudney worked for three days, treating an endless stream of casualties arriving at the CCS. At the end of the third day the old hop-house grew dark and cold, like a cave, and the voices of the medical staff and cries of the wounded echoed up into the eaves. Wherever the lanterns that were strung up along the beams threw their light, Doudney could see blood, splashed up the walls and soaked into the strings of dried hops still hanging from the beams. He would now always think of blood when he saw garlands of hops, not of harvest festivals. He was aching and exhausted, his spirits low. But then the patient on the stretcher in front of him recognised the padre: he had been one of his parishioners in Bath. They chatted briefly, exchanging the little local news that each had from letters home, and Doudney cleaned and dressed his wounds. He started to feel more cheerful, healed by the man on the stretcher.

Finally it was his turn to sleep and he stumbled to the small cot set up for him in a corridor. He was woken several hours later by the sound of engines and went out to the driveway to see who had arrived. It was the medics of the field ambulance, who were also stationed in the hop-house. They had been working in aid posts at the front for days on end, and Doudney could see the exhaustion crushing them as they climbed down from the vehicles. They walked towards the hop-store to treat the wounded waiting there, but Doudney stopped them: get some sleep, he told them, then have breakfast, and then go back to work. Grey but grateful faces turned towards him. If the padre says so, he knows best.

Doudney and the other chaplains were coming to understand something very important: someone needed to tell medics when they had worked long or hard enough. Their work at medical posts and hospitals all over the front was earning the padres a very particular authority. Medical staff came to trust them implicitly, so when men like Doudney or Abbott told them to rest, sleep, eat or pray, they did as they were told. Telling them that they had worked enough became the most important and useful thing that chaplains could do at their post. They looked out for the nurse with dark circles under her eyes. They showed the surgeon working during a battle his red and swollen hands, and told him to get some rest.[13] They waited up for medical staff working late and made sure there was some warm dinner for them, keeping them company while they ate. There was an MO who manned an aid post entirely on his own, night after night, in case casualties crawled in from the dark battlefield. When his chaplain heard about it, he took a chess set and joined the officer in his dugout every night, the two men playing games and listening out for the cries of the wounded.[14]

As summer ended and work at the CCS slowed, Doudney got a chance to explore the place. He was particularly fascinated by the laboratory run by a young Scottish chemist, John Annan, full of the latest microscopes, with sterilisation equipment steaming and bubbling across the wooden tabletops. He befriended Annan, and the scientist called the padre to the lab whenever he found something particularly exciting under his lens. But Doudney also thought about how to improve life at the CCS. He wrote to his parishioners at home, asking for a gramophone and records so that he could play music in the convalescent wards. They obliged with whatever he asked for, and in return he filled his letters to them with exciting descriptions of his 'nerve-shaking times up at the front', telling them about aeroplanes, captive balloons and the variety of guns. His parishioners in Bath even donated a motorcycle, which he used to go up the line to hold funerals.[15]

As the days went by, the convalescent wards were gradually emptying, and by October there were almost no patients left at the station. Doudney's work now mostly consisted of burying the dead. On 13 October, he was asked to a nearby cemetery to oversee the service for eight dead soldiers. There was a lorry going that way, so Doudney didn't take his motorcycle, being happy to catch a lift. The other passenger was a medical officer who was pleased to have the padre along for the ride as he was good company. There wasn't enough space in the front cab for the driver and his two passengers to sit next to each other, so Doudney sat on the floor with his legs dangling out of the door to give the tired medic more room. He chatted about his favourite topic, wireless telegraphy and radiography, and asked the medic about his own work, so time passed without the men really noticing the shells falling not far off.

Suddenly a shell burst right in front of the vehicle, covering it in mud and slamming it to a violent halt. When the MO clambered out of the cab he saw immediately that the driver and the padre had been injured, but the three men managed to take cover behind the wall of a ruined house. Doudney insisted that the doctor first examine the driver, who had been wounded in the thigh, but the MO knew with one look that the injuries to the padre's back and stomach were far more serious. As the shelling continued, Doudney begged him to leave and take the driver back to the medical post, but the MO was having none of it. Finally the fire stopped for

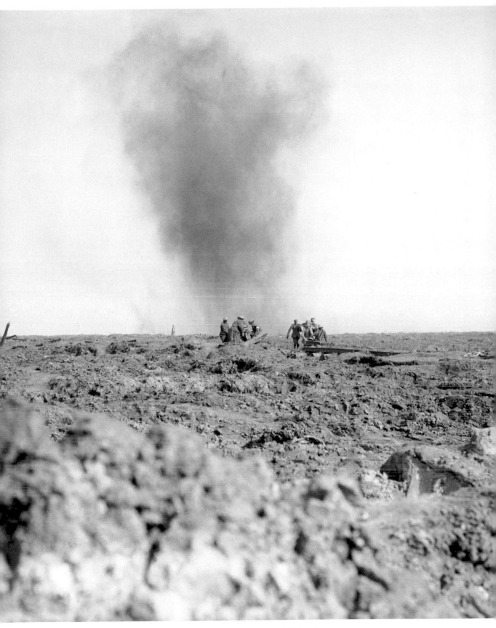

Stretcher bearers on a carry from the battlefield during the Somme.
The photograph was taken from a forward trench and shows a shell exploding
in the distance as the bearers work deep in no-man's-land.

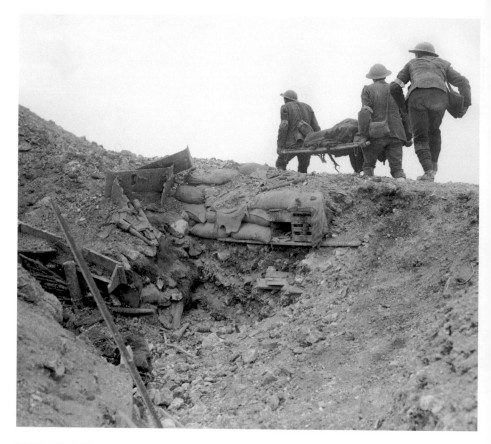

(*Above*) Stretcher bearers carry a wounded man around the edge of a collapsed trench.

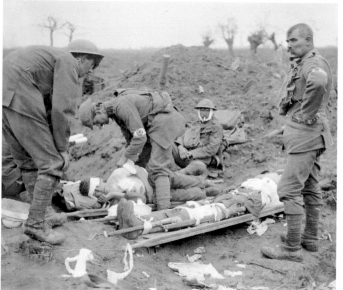

(*Left*) In trenches to the rear, bearers treat two soldiers with multiple wounds. They use dressings to prevent bleeding, and have improvised wooden splints to hold fractured limbs in place. They are observed by a 'walking' case who has his head bandaged to contain a wound to his jaw.

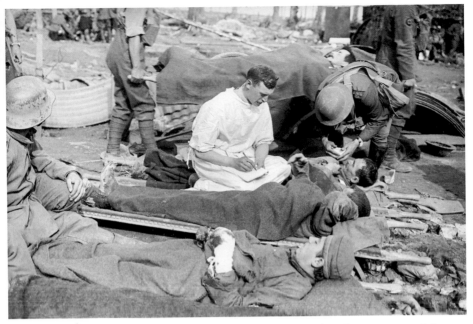

(*Above*) The doc and the padre (*in tin helmet*) tending to British and German wounded.

(*Below*) Wounded as far as the eye can see awaiting removal on the Menin Road, September 1917. One motorised ambulance has become stuck in the mud. In front of it is a heap of stretchers.

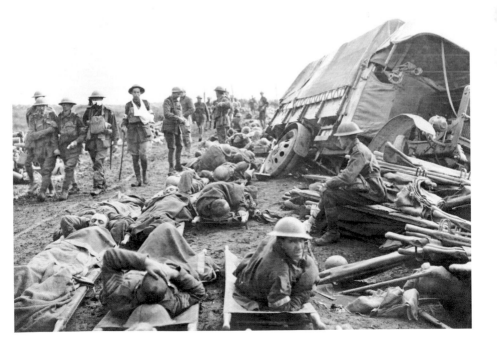

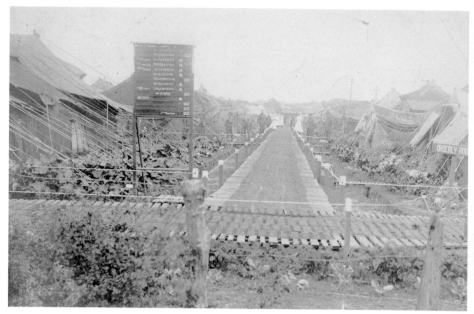

(*Above*) No. 44 Casualty Clearing Station at Puchevillers, where Norman Pritchard served as a surgeon. No. 44 was so large it required significant signage to enable its staff to find their way around the hundreds of tents that comprised the various medical departments.

(*Below*) Some of the staff at No. 44 in a photograph taken in the CCS vegetable garden.

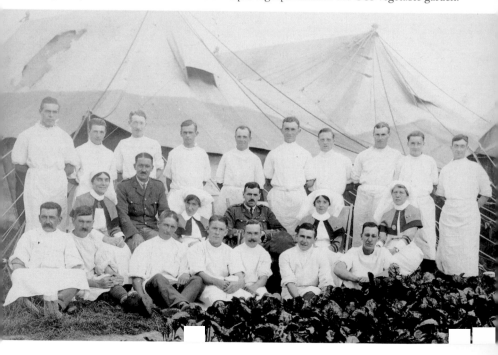

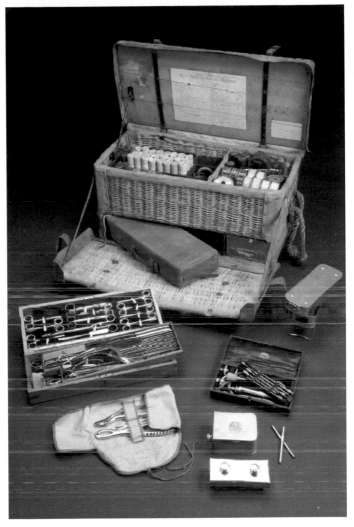

(*Right*) A field ambulance medical kit with a full set of sharps, similar to one used by Geoffrey Hardwick of the 59th Field Ambulance.

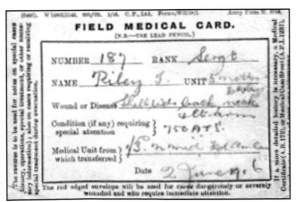

(*Left*) The Field Medical Card of Sgt Thomas Riley. On 2 June 1916 Sgt Riley was wounded in his back, neck and left arm. Despite this, he was patched up and sent back to his battalion in time for 'the big push'. He was killed on the first day of the Somme.

(*Right*) Interior of a British 'Khaki' ambulance train. Specially built, the train had electric lighting, wide aisles to enable nursing and stretchers and hanging straps for the patients in the top bunks to steady themselves during bumpy journeys, Doullens, 27 April 1918

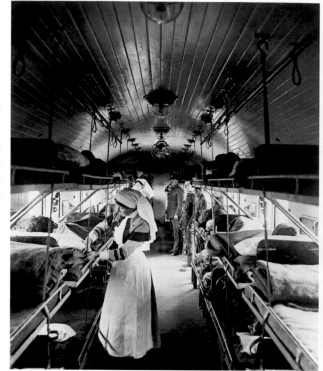

(*Below*) Orderlies entraining a patient wounded during the early months of Passchendaele, August 1917.

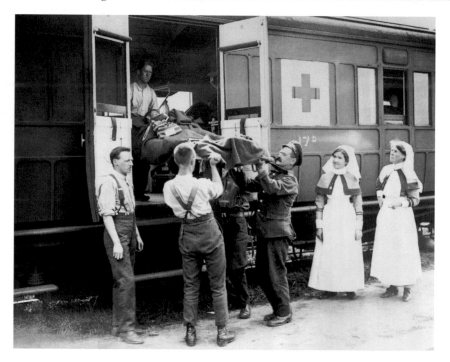

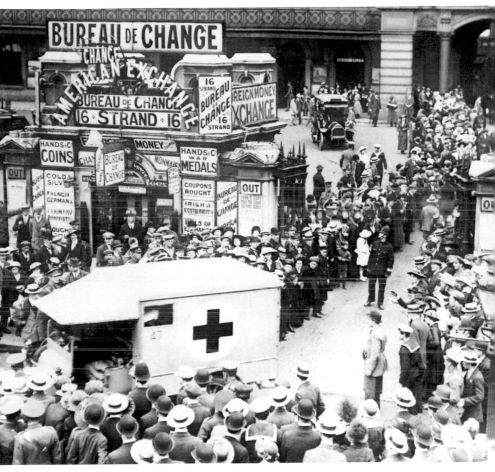

Crowds throng Charing Cross Station to cheer casualties from the Battle of the Somme as they are transported by members of the London Ambulance Column to hospitals around London, 8 July 1916.

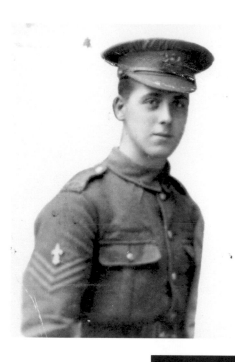

(*Left*) The wounded: Bert Payne.

(*Below*) The padre: Charles Doudney.

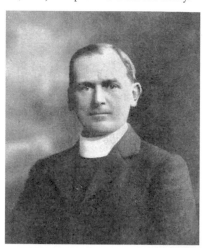

(*Right*) The medic:
Charles McKerrow

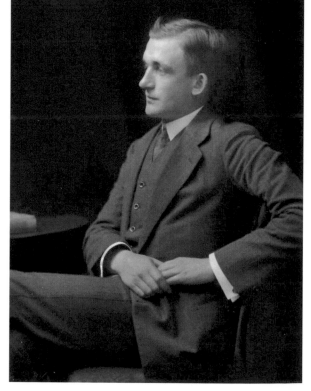

long enough for the lorry to hurtle back to the CCS. News had already reached the CO, who had sent for Anthony Bowlby, the most senior surgeon on the entire front. Staff gathered in groups outside the operating theatre, nervously pacing around and pleading with the Almighty to save the padre. But his wounds were too severe and Doudney died on the operating table.

He was buried on the morning of 20 October 1915, with a beautiful sun breaking through the Flanders mist and heavy guns booming in the distance. The staff of the CCS had seen many men die over the last year, but no loss of life had affected them as badly as that of Charles Doudney.[16] And no one missed him more than his friend John Annan, who had so enjoyed the chaplain's company and the many conversations they had in the laboratory. He wrote to Doudney's widow and asked for a photograph of the padre. She sent him one and he propped it up amongst the microscopes and steamers, to remind him of his friend.

Chaplain John Murray was forty-seven years old when he arrived in France from St Paul's, Walworth, a parish in one of East London's most deprived boroughs. It was early 1917, and it had taken Murray a while to get the posting. He was initially rejected because of his age, but he pestered the Bishop of London, who finally gave way. Yet when the job came, it wasn't what Murray had hoped for. Rather than being sent to the front line to serve with a battalion, he was to be chaplain to the 8th General Hospital in Rouen. It didn't feel like being in a war: it was the sort of posting he could have got at home. When his wife watched him pack his suitcase she saw that he included his sketchbook and pastels. Monet had painted the cathedral after all, and perhaps he would get a chance to do some drawing too, which would make up for not being too busy.

When Murray disembarked at Rouen, it seemed to him that the entire town had become a hospital. The station was full of hospital trains, the air thick with the smell of blood and the stench of gas still lingering in some of the soldiers' clothes, and on the platform he had to pick his way through a tangle of men and stretchers waiting to be moved. In the streets there seemed to be no vehicles other than queues of canvas-backed ambulances on their way to one of the huge base hospitals that had taken over many of the town's larger buildings. As he walked to No. 8, Murray passed few pedestrians who weren't uniformed nurses hurrying along with parcels under their arms, or bandaged soldiers walking slowly on the arms of comrades, wearing patched uniforms with the shadows of hastily laundered bloodstains still upon them. Yet it still didn't feel like war to Murray; it was too far away from the guns and the courage of men under fire.

At the hospital, a huge converted hotel, someone pointed Murray in the general direction of his accommodation. His room was large and comfortable – he would have preferred the mud of a dugout – and he was sharing it with two doctors. Later that night they came off-duty and introduced themselves: Fergusson was the hospital's radiographer and Armstrong the pathologist. They seemed pleased to see him and the next evening he found out why: there was nothing the two doctors liked more than a good philosophical debate about God and the war. He tried to be tactful in his replies: their white coats and exhausted faces were testament to the day's hardships and gave them an authority that he felt he was lacking. But he hadn't come to France for discussions about philosophy. He wrote to his wife that he feared for his spiritual life at the hospital and that he was praying for guidance. After a week in Rouen he thought he had utterly failed in making himself useful.[17]

But Murray was a practical man and after a while his wife noticed from his letters that his mood was picking up. He had begun to find ways to be useful. It wasn't just the official tasks of a chaplain – ward visits, Sunday services and burials, and helping out with letter writing – that gave him a sense of purpose. He was thinking about what else was needed. Helping the patients with their letters, he suddenly realised that there was no one in the hospital whose responsibility it was to deliver the post. It was haphazardly done by a nurse or orderly, if there was time. So Murray became the hospital postman, trotting round with the mail every morning and afternoon, delivering letters to the wards, offices and nurses' quarters. Soon he got to know everyone in the hospital, patients and staff alike, and they got to know him too. Everyone was pleased to see the padre who brought them their post and soon his days were filled with chatting to people and passing on hospital news.

After several weeks as postman Murray probably knew his way around the building better than anyone else and had come to admire the place. It was well equipped, with dedicated staff; it even had one of the new mental wards.[18] He was proud of being part of it, but felt that he hadn't yet earned his position. So one night, before his room-mates had a chance to start another debate about the will of God, he asked if they would help him pick up some basic medical education. The doctors looked at each other. Why not? The padre was a decent sort, and they really enjoyed their late-night discussions with him, which helped them calm down after a day's work. They were happy to oblige and drew up a curriculum. Each of them would tutor the padre individually whenever they had a spare moment, so he had to be ready when they were.

Several days later, the course began. Murray had just returned from holding funerals for several hours, when Armstrong turned up at his office with a steel theatre dish. Today was 'abnormal liver' day, he explained, and since the padre was such a keen artist, how about he painted it, and Armstrong would explain what had gone wrong with the liver as he went along. The padre hurried to get out his sketchbook and pastels and began to draw the organ, as the doctor leaned over his shoulder, detailing symptoms, treatment and cause of death. When he had finished, Armstrong reviewed Murray's drawing. It was pretty good for a first go, but he hadn't got the colour and texture of the pus quite right. It was the paints, Murray explained: a cheap box, not up to the job; and the paper was all wrong. The next day he bought expensive paints,

sable brushes and a proper artist's pad, and in the hospital workshop built himself an easel for future classes. But he didn't just
use his paints for anatomical pictures. When he received a letter
from the father of a dead soldier asking for a description of his
son's grave, Murray sent him a perfect sketch.

For all the ways he had found to make himself useful at No.
8, Murray still longed for a front-line posting and bombarded the
relevant officials with letters begging to be reassigned. In the
meantime it seemed sensible to prepare for the move by acquiring
the knowledge and skills that he would most need at the front.
When the first waves of casualties arrived from the battle of Arras,
he was assigned to escort the walking wounded from the ambulances to their wards because he knew the way better than anyone.
He used these journeys, some of them painfully slow, to question
the men about conditions at the front and the kinds of injuries
they had seen. He also got himself put on stretcher-bearer duty,
unloading casualties from the ambulances and carrying them up
the steps into the hospital. Even this relatively short trip was
physically exhausting and, after the first day, Murray fell into bed,
his arms, shoulders and back aching. But even more draining was
seeing the state of the wounded. For the first time he saw men
who had been brought straight from the battlefield, having
received little or no medical care and covered in so much mud
that he could barely tell they were human, let alone man or officer,
their faces unshaven, grey and hollow-eyed.

Murray also learned to tailor his religious activities to the needs
of the hospital. He tried for a regular service, but it proved impossible, so he focused mostly on giving Communion to the patients
on the wards – small, private ceremonies at each bed. One morning
he arrived on a ward that was full of casualties, with the busy
staff running back and forth. Careful not to get in their way, he
started to unpack his Communion box, when behind him he heard
a strained, hoarse whisper asking if anyone could help. In a bed
nearby Murray found a soldier who had been so badly burned
that his entire head was wrapped in a mass of bandages. Two

small holes had been cut in the dressings for his eyes and another for his mouth, and blood drops from his wounds were starting to fleck the clean white dressing.

Murray asked the man if he could help, trying not to be shocked by his desperate black eyes. When he bent down to make out the patient's words he noticed that in place of his lips there was just raw flesh. He was thirsty, whispered the soldier, so thirsty. There was lemonade in a jug at the end of the ward and Murray fetched it. The soldier had a beaker and a straw on his bedside table, so the padre poured the drink into it and eased the straw into the soldier's mouth as gently as he could. The man was too weak to sit up to take the drink, so Murray put his arm under the soldier's shoulder to support him. Even through the pyjamas and bandaging Murray could feel the heat of his burned body. The soldier drank for a little while and then lay back. Murray sat by him and, when the wounded man was ready for more, helped him up again and fed the straw through the hole in the bandages. Finally the soldier had finished and whispered his thanks. As he closed his swollen eyelids to go to sleep, Murray returned to his set and packed it up. He had given an unexpected form of Communion in the ward that day.

At the end of May 1917 came the front-line posting he had longed for: Murray was to report to the 12th and 13th Battalions of the Royal Sussex regiment, which was to defend British positions at Passchendaele. Murray was sorry to leave the hospital, but he felt he was now ready to be at the sharp end of the war. Yet there were still things he had no experience of. On the march to the front he asked the sergeant if he could carry one of the soldiers' packs for a while, to see how it felt. The sergeant was reluctant to let an untrained older man carry a bulky, 100-pound pack. But Murray insisted and the sergeant handed him his own, assuring him it was as heavy as any in the battalion. Murray marched for four miles before handing it back. The new padre was a bit strange, word went through the ranks. Strange, but probably all right.

On 31 July 1917 Murray helped the MO set up a medical post

as the Sussexes were thrown into battle. For the first hour they tried to clear the area of the kit abandoned by advancing men: everywhere Murray looked he saw mountains of packs, rations and abandoned bicycles. But there wasn't time to sort it all out before the first casualties arrived, and by lunchtime they had dressed the wounds of 530 men. They had also run out of bearers and Murray organised a group of POWs to help out. But this still wasn't enough, and with so many broken men waiting for help in the shell holes, Murray put himself on bearer duty.

On the battlefield he soon found a wounded man and then, luckily, a bearer team to carry him back, but not before the casualty had clutched his sleeve and begged him to find his mate, somewhere out there, badly hurt. Follow the blood, Padre, you've got to find him. One of the bearers agreed to go with Murray, but following a single blood trail on the field of Passchendaele was impossible. They crouched close to the ground, looking for clues, listening out for moans and cries. Then the bearer was hit, not seriously, but badly enough for Murray to send him back to the aid post. As he continued on alone he suddenly heard a faint cry from one of the shell holes and broke into a run, waving back at the bearer to show him where he was heading. Then, climbing down into the hole, he found the soldier's mate.

The wounded man was in a bad state and Murray crouched down to examine his wounds. They weren't immediately life-threatening, but he knew he would never get the man back on his own. Then he carefully stood up to see where he was. The firing had moved away from them, so at least they were in no immediate danger. But it was starting to rain heavily, from dark, surging clouds. Murray dragged canvas and boards over their shell hole to make a roof. The rain saturated his tunic as he worked. When he had finished and crawled into the improvised shelter, the wounded man pointed into one corner. Murray hadn't noticed the dead soldier lying there, killed in that morning's fighting. He got up again and dragged the body out of the shelter. He would attend to him later. For now he had to care for the living.

By three o'clock in the afternoon the rain had turned the battlefield into a quagmire and water was streaming into their shelter. The injured man was growing frightened, not just from his wounds, but from the cold and the wet and the strangeness of the battlefield. Murray asked him if there was anything else he could do. Would the padre sing him a hymn? So, after a short prayer, Murray started to sing. For hours he sang every hymn he could remember, softly and accompanied by the rain battering on the canvas above. After a while the injured man calmed visibly. Several times he asked Murray for 'Abide with Me' as the eventide fell. Finally, at around eight o'clock, Murray heard voices outside their shelter and got up to wave over a team of bearers.

The next day Murray worked alongside the MO in the aid post. He never left the dugout, pausing only to catch glimpses of bearers struggling towards them in the mud. On 2 August, the third day of Passchendaele, British forces retook positions they had lost earlier in the back-and-forth of battle, and the MO was summoned to go forward with them. He left Murray in charge of the aid post and, together with five dressers, the padre worked all day. Then the guns turned back towards them. The queue of men outside had attracted the attention of the enemy and the post was hit by a shell. Murray remembered little of the next few hours, when he was dug out of the mud and taken to the nearest CCS with serious concussion.

He spent the next six weeks recuperating in England, nursed at home by his wife. But by the end of September he was back with the Sussexes, and nothing seemed to have changed. The battle was grinding on, with no sign of a winner, and the mud still covered everything and everyone. He was comforted to see that the men had missed him, but distraught at how many of them were dead. One day, when out on the battlefield to retrieve the wounded, he found five fresh corpses, so he stopped and began to dig a grave for them. Preoccupied with this work, he didn't notice that the firing was getting ever closer, until a bearer managed to drag him away. What use was a dead padre to anyone? It was the living who needed him most.

At the end of September, Murray was back with the MO running a new aid post as the battalion took part in the Polygon Wood offensive to take the main ridge east of Ypres. The post was one of the busiest of the battle, although it was doing very little real medical work. Instead it acted as a clearing post: 3,000 walking wounded were processed there in the first twelve hours of the battle. Murray and the MO worked in tandem, with the MO assessing the casualties and the padre logging them and filling out the wounded label as the MO dictated. It was mind-numbing work. Another chaplain arrived to see if he could help. Yet when Murray found him a chair and a pile of logbooks, the man left in a huff, saying he hadn't come to the Western Front to be a clerk. Murray shook his head as he watched him go. As a padre, you did whatever was necessary – digging, carrying, clerking. During a short break the MO came over to his table as Murray shook out his arm, which had stiffened from writing. He was sorry to have given his colleague such a mundane job, the doctor said, but at this moment it was the most useful thing he could possibly be doing.

Early gains at Polygon Wood led to misplaced optimism about the imminent collapse of the German forces at Passchendaele. The Sussexes fought on until late October, when the High Command finally called a halt to the offensive. But the work didn't stop at Murray's aid post. When three soldiers sheltering nearby were hit by a shell and killed, Murray went out to try and bury them. It was almost impossible to dig a grave in the mud, which slid back as soon as he removed his spade. As he sweated to make some kind of grave, he suddenly noticed the MO digging alongside him – a small return for all the help the padre had given him. Together they buried the men as best they could, and Murray pronounced the Committal. As the two men walked back to the aid post they realised they were both covered in mud from head to foot. In the end – doctor or padre, friend or enemy – everyone looked the same at Passchendaele.

In December, Murray received orders to return home. The

Sussexes were truly sorry to see him go and held a farewell concert in his honour at which they presented him with a cigarette case, engraved by one of the soldiers who was a silversmith. He had finally had the war that he wanted. He had come to understand what war meant for the men who fought in it and for those who tried to save their lives. He wrote home to his wife with some satisfaction that he felt he had, after all, been able to serve with something approaching a quiet conscience.

Many of the chaplains caring for the wounded at the Western Front found great satisfaction in their work – some even discovered real joy.[19] But for Cyril Horsley-Smith, formerly of a rural Norfolk parish and now chaplain to the 1/5th Battalion London Regiment, his days at the front held no fulfilment or happiness. He knew what his duties were and he was certain of one thing: a chaplain's real work was not to bring in the wounded. There were men who could do that job much better than he could. He had come to the front to give Communion, lead prayers and bury the dead. He didn't need to look for something to do when he was posted to a CCS; he knew what was required of him.

No. 7 Casualty Clearing Station was located near Melville and, although it was some distance away from the front, Horsley-Smith found it to be a terrible place. From his first day there, he felt it was exacting a toll on him from which he might never recover. As he took no interest in the medical work, he made no friends among the doctors and nurses. He strongly objected to the presence of female staff at the CCS, who – he felt – should not be made to witness such dreadful suffering. If he himself felt the strain so keenly, what must it be like for the nurses? He kept himself separate from the staff and, when he wasn't visiting patients or fulfilling his religious duties, stayed in his tent.

There was plenty of chaplaincy work for him to do. He held daily morning services and led prayers in the evening. On Sundays he was robed almost all day, regardless of the size of the congregation. Yet although he preached devotion and consolation, he

himself didn't find any in his work at No. 7. He had also been
forced to take on one additional job – that of censoring the men's
letters. It had become a common duty for padres: no one else
had the time, and the men generally preferred it that their letters
were read by the chaplain rather than the officers. It was a boring
and time-consuming activity, and for Horsley-Smith it seemed
almost deliberately designed to emphasise the pointlessness of
his ministry at the front. Reading for hours at a time in the dim
light of his tent, the endless pages of soldier scrawl were undeni-
able evidence of the men's ignorance and godlessness and of his
inability to reach them.

Yet it was his real work that gave him the greatest cause for
despair. Several times each day he gathered what little strength he
had left to make his way to the huge moribund ward. He could
have recognised the ward even with his eyes closed. Moribund wards
were all but silent: they had none of the chatter of the ordinary
wounded wards, just low levels of moaning and the occasional gasp
of pain. Every time he got to the entrance of the large tent he
faltered for a second and then braced himself to go in. As far as
Horsley-Smith was concerned, death had an unrelenting grip on
No. 7 CCS: it had a 50 per cent mortality rate – high even by the
grim standards of the Western Front. For many here the chaplain's
visit represented the last stage of their lives. Gripping his Bible until
his knuckles were white, Horsley-Smith walked into the ward,
knowing he would need to comfort every man there, one after the
other. He tried to give consolation and absolution to the grey-faced
soldiers who often seemed to be vanishing before his very eyes,
some whispering, others barely breathing. Often he couldn't even
tell the living from the dead. For the chaplain there was very little
healing at No. 7 – it was all about dying.

He received letters from the families of the men he had absolved
and noticed that, in many cases, the death of their loved one had
come as a complete shock. Should they have been warned, very
gently, of the patient's deteriorating condition? But how to find
out who was close to the end? He could have talked to the nurses,

but he was reluctant to have any more than the minimum of contact with them, and he didn't have enough medical knowledge to understand the patient charts. So he devised his own system during his nightly rounds of the ward. He would stop by each bed and lightly touch, with the palm of his hand, the nose of the patient sleeping there. If their nose was very cold, he knew the end could not be far away, and he would write that very night to the man's family to prepare them. Horsley-Smith was almost always right. Night after night he made his inspections, walking carefully and quietly in the dark around each bed in the ward, his hand outstretched; and each cold touch to his hand filled him with dread. Only once did a soldier wake as Horsley-Smith's palm touched his nose. Sitting up, he swore at the padre: 'This bugger says I'm going to die.' He wasn't going to die, he shouted, waking the other patients. Then he sank back and, with his eyes still on the padre, he died.

A full moribund ward meant many burials, and the thought of more funerals was often too much for Horsley-Smith. One thing above all came to symbolise death for him and the other chaplains: the brown army blanket.[20] Once, midway through a funeral service, he realised how short the bag was in the grave in front of him. He continued with the ceremony, but soon worked out that he was burying a man who had been torn in half. Another chaplain was called to perform a funeral service and realised that it was for the entire bearer team with whom he had been working. Fifteen men lay before him wrapped in brown blankets, fifteen men with whom he had spent months carrying in the mud.[21]

But it wasn't just the strain of endlessly repeating the Committal that got to Horsley-Smith. There was also the plain terror of the trip from No. 7 CCS to the Noeux-les-Mines cemetery a few miles away. The padre joined orderlies and sanitation squads in the cab of the lorry carrying the dead, and on their way they had to pass a crossroads that was almost constantly shelled by the enemy. The trick was for the driver to accelerate as the lorry approached the junction and cross it at full speed. Horsley-Smith dreaded the journey that he was forced to make several times a week, never knowing if he would get back to the CCS alive. But at the cemetery he gathered himself and conducted ceremonies that always impressed the bearers and drivers with their thorough, unhurried respect. He carefully recorded each man's name, dates and the location of his grave for the bereaved families and the authorities. Then he packed away his equipment and surplice and tried not to think about the journey home as he walked reluctantly back to the waiting lorry.

And so it was for the remainder of Chaplain Horsley-Smith's war. There was no joy or fulfilment, just dread and fear and the cold touch of death on his hand, night after night. After the war he remembered only the eyes of the men about to die, and the faces of the dead. But although he hated and feared every single minute he spent on the Western Front, he continued with his duties and spared himself nothing. It never occurred to him that he could have requested a position to the rear. He was doing his real work, and there was no one else who could do it.

In the last months of the war he received a letter from a brother chaplain. He had ministered recently to a soldier who had once been a patient in Horsley-Smith's moribund ward, but had survived. The soldier had specifically asked the chaplain to find Horsley-Smith and pass on his thanks for all the kindnesses he had shown him at No. 7 CCS. He had been a real brother to him, day after day, helping him forward, never giving up. He was alive because of the sombre, lonely chaplain and his brave dedication to his real work.

Chaplain Montagu Bere took up his new post at No. 43 Casualty Clearing Station just before Easter 1916. He would see out three Holy Weeks on the Western Front and it was only there that he felt he really came to understand the true meaning of the Passion. Battles always seemed to be hardest at Easter, and the wards were full of suffering men. His first Good Friday, 21 April 1916, came during the battle of Verdun, and Bere was struggling to keep up with the men who needed his ministry. He gave Communion in a ward so full that stretchers were lying between the beds and all along the central aisle, so he had to pick his way carefully from man to man. When he had finished, he looked around to see where he should go next. Then he saw a scene he would never forget – as if a devotional painting had come to life before his eyes. Amongst the tangled bloodstained sheets, a great broken man lay in the arms of an exhausted-looking nurse, hair escaping from her white scarf, who looked down on him murmuring words of calm and pity, while a doctor in a gore-stained apron removed huge pieces of shrapnel from the man's flesh. Bere could see the metal shards in his wounds and the man shuddering in agony as they were pulled out.

A friendly and practical man, Bere had been a curate for sixteen years in a Docklands parish in London and had seen plenty of hardship. No. 43 CCS had already had a couple of Anglicans and a Roman Catholic chaplain, so when Bere arrived, staff expected him to hold a service to introduce himself – and then probably not do much else. But Bere wasn't like his predecessors. He was sharing a tent with some of the MOs and, instead of announcing his first service, he set out to build some bookshelves and bedside tables for them all, making use of some packing cases he had found. Within a day or two of his arrival the tent was fully furnished. By that time he had also fixed the broken stove in the mess anteroom, without being asked.

It soon became standard practice at No. 43 to seek out the padre if a job needed doing and there was no one designated to do it. Bere spoke fluent French, so he accompanied the quartermaster into town to negotiate with the local suppliers. When French or Belgian luminaries came to inspect the CCS, it was Bere who walked them round the wards, laboratories and X-ray facilities. His carpentry skills were in great demand: he repaired everything from broken stretchers to the roofs of the wooden huts. When he discovered some old deckchairs, he repaired the frames and sewed new canvas backs for them, before proudly laying them out in front of the nurses' tents so that they could sunbathe in comfort. And when one of the matrons noticed that the padre could sew, she asked him whether he would help out in the linen store occasionally. Soon Bere found himself doing nothing but sewing for weeks at a time, name-taping the sheets, pillow cases and blankets that were washed at a local laundry. Then torn uniforms and unravelling socks were added to his pile, and Bere sewed and darned until his eyes and fingers were too sore to continue or the wind blew out the candle in his tent.

He turned a small patch of land at the back of the CCS into a garden, where he grew vegetables and flowers and kept a few chickens. The chickens occasionally escaped from their coop, and the padre could be seen chasing them – once all the way into a ward, where one of the birds flew into the Sister's headdress. The chaplain apologised profusely before hurrying from the ward, a chicken under each arm. By now he was also in charge of the payroll and the mess accounts, and he was getting so good with the French suppliers that one of them had tipped him in chocolate, which he turned into an evening's worth of good cocoa for the nurses. And if that wasn't enough, he even learned cobbling, so that he could mend the soldiers' boots. When he returned the repaired and polished pairs to the wards, their owners were surprised to see that they had been mended by the man who also prayed with them.

In June 1916 the commanding officer received instructions to integrate the CCS into the forthcoming offensive. They were one of the units closest to the front line and would be used as both aid post and hospital ward. There was a lot that needed doing in preparation, and by now it was simply assumed that the padre would be part of it. As truck after truck turned into the CCS driveway, Bere spent several days unloading tons of extra medical supplies, stretchers and linen. They were sent a consignment of temporary Armstrong huts, which they put up under the padre's supervision, and after he had helped lay paths to the new huts and tents, he began to dig a trench for a water pipe so that a new water tank could be set up. Thus Bere spent much of June outside and there was activity everywhere he looked. Aside from the endless stream of lorries, which sounded like rush-hour traffic on the Bayswater Road, squadrons of aircraft flew back and forth overhead, and guns were test-fired. There was so much noise around them that when the CCS's staff held a cricket match, no one could hear the ball strike the bat.

When he looked back, Bere could remember giving only one short religious service during the entire time. But he had other priorities. The previous year at Verdun he had been pitifully unable to help the MOs and the nurses. Now, like other padres at the front, he asked to be given some basic medical training. Soon he moved from tent to tent, watching the doctors, nurses and orderlies, taking notes and finishing his rounds in the surgical wards, where the surgeons tried to prepare him for what was to come.

On 1 July the barrage that thundered up and down the front woke up the staff at the CCS. They strained to hear how the battle was going, and some of them reckoned they could hear the whistles and shouts as the men went over the top. But not long afterwards, as Bere waited outside the admissions tent, he began to hear something else – a shuffling, dragging sound, broken by cries and moans. Coming towards him was a column of walking wounded: hundreds of men, the lame leading the blind, all covered in blood, their uniforms ragged, their faces white with shock. Bere and the orderlies rushed towards them to help them into the tent. Soon afterwards the first bearer teams arrived, all of them grim-faced, speechless, horror-struck at what they had seen. As he sat down one of the many casualties that he would carry that day, one bearer broke the cardinal rule of never swearing in front of the padre, as he tried to describe what he had witnessed. 'A bloody mug's game,' he mumbled.[22]

It would be one of the longest days of Bere's life. He ran from tent to tent, helping wherever he was needed. He dressed wounds, carried men into theatre, prayed with the dying and performed all the other jobs that nobody seemed to have time for. He found the patients new clothing if their uniforms had been torn to pieces. He brought them drawstring bags and carefully stored their valuables as they watched, before taking down their details and promising to write to their families that very night.

By the evening he realised that they had been working all day without a break, so he went to the kitchens and made soup and sandwiches. Putting it all on a trolley, he went round the wards and operating theatres and insisted that the medical staff stop, just for a few minutes, and have something to eat. Some MOs had been working so hard that their hands were swollen or blistered and he had to call a nurse to tend them. Then a bearer came to tell Bere that the newly dug cemetery nearby was full, so could he come and hold a funeral service? After checking identity tags and making sure that personal possessions had all been removed and safely stored, he stood in the night and called the Committal against the thunder of shellfire in the distance. Then he went to his tent to write all the letters he had promised, for the living.

The second day was much the same. Bere helped wherever he was needed and his presence provided a small degree of calm for both soldiers and staff. On the third day a column of wounded German POWs arrived at the CCS. As Bere was the only one at the station who could speak German (in addition to his French), he was put in charge of admitting them to a separate guarded hut. It took him hours to record the name and number of each German soldier and translate the doctor's diagnosis into the logbook. They all wanted him to contact their families, and he tried to explain that he would as soon as he had time. But he made sure that he spent as much time comforting them as writing down their details.

And so it went on. By 6 July the pressure had started to ease a little and Bere finally found time to write to his wife. There had been fewer funerals than he expected: the surgeons had done excellent work. They had already moved some of their patients onto hospital trains heading for base hospitals or England, so there were now a few empty beds. They had one special ward for patients who were too seriously wounded to be moved, and Bere spent as much time there as he could. Several of them were Londoners and they reminded him of home. He was particularly fond of a butcher's boy from Putney who had been all but torn apart. Bere brought him into the operating theatre every day and waited outside to return him to his ward when the surgeons had finished.

And while he was waiting he made himself useful. The men awaiting surgery in the pre-operative tent were terrified: anaesthetics were primitive and they could hear the screams of men being operated on in theatre. Bere comforted them, saying special prayers if they wished, chatting with them or just holding their hands. Then he went to the post-operative ward and waited for the men to come round. One afternoon a nurse found the padre gently supporting a patient while he cried and vomited after his operation. 'We treat you like a batman, Padre,' she called over to him. Bere looked up and smiled. There was no bigger compliment.

When the butcher's boy was finally stable enough to be moved on, he asked if Bere would accompany him to the station. For the first time the padre saw the chaos at the railheads and he stayed for a long time, fetching water and food for the wounded on their stretchers, kneeling by their side to soothe their nerves or say a prayer. The railhead now became his second parish and he spent as much time on the platform as he could. He helped the orderlies to load the train, until the last man was safely on board. Then, as it pulled slowly out of the station, he was often the last man the wounded could see on the platform, waving them off.

Bere got to know the station and its staff so well that it soon fell to him to meet trains with patients arriving from the front and organise their transport to the CCS, either as a long column of walking wounded that he would escort or on stretchers in ambulances. The stationmaster let him use his office while he waited for trains. There the hollow chime of the bell, which the station staff had built for their clock out of huge shell casings, reminded him of his church back home, providing some comfort while he waited in the dark.

It was months before he began to perform regular religious services. But Bere knew that his other acts of service for the men in his care were just as important. He worried that he didn't make much impact on those without faith, so he welcomed any kind of religious devotion wherever he found it. Unlike other padres, Bere was happy to listen to a wounded man tell him of his vision of angels appearing above no-man's-land: if it kept the man alive, that was good enough for him. There was talk of a National Mission to convert the soldiers at the front, but Bere thought it was conceived by men who knew nothing of the realities of war. He was furious with an orderly who belonged to the Salvation Army and preached to a captive audience in the surgical ward. A hospital ward full of broken men, some of them barely alive, was no place to try and make conversions.

When Bere gave Communion in the ward, the men in the nearby beds went quiet – and even if they didn't participate in the ceremony, they usually stubbed out their cigarettes. One time he had asked a patient what his religion was, and the man replied 'trench feet'. Bere had laughed, much to the surprise – and approval – of everyone within earshot. He had been deeply moved when, during one of his services, he saw a man whose legs had been shot away holding a hymn book for a soldier who had lost his arms, both of them entirely focused on singing.

When winter arrived, the battle of the Somme already felt like a distant memory at No. 43 CCS. Bere cooked Christmas dinner in the staff mess, supplemented by parcels from his wife. That winter was especially cold, and most mornings the staff saw the padre pushing a wheeled trolley out into the forest to gather wood to make charcoal. In return for all his services, the surgeons invited him into theatre to watch them operate on particularly interesting cases. His medical knowledge had increased hugely and was becoming useful. He advised his wife when she became an early victim of the Spanish flu, and when she told him that a neighbour was suspected of having died of cerebrospinal fever (a form of meningitis), his reply revealed his expertise. He didn't think a culture had been taken from the man's spinal fluid, he wrote. Here in France, if there was the least doubt about a diagnosis, sputum or blood was sent to a bacteriologist. No decent doctor would fail to have a culture grown when there was any doubt as to the exact bacillus causing the complaint, he concluded.

Spring of 1917 came late, so there was little Bere could do in his garden. But there were plenty of other tasks. A POW camp had opened nearby and Bere had been asked to conduct services in German. Where there are human beings, there is work for a priest, he wrote to his wife. He had managed to find a German Bible, but printed up German hymn sheets himself. He spent many hours at the camp, holding services and writing letters for the prisoners; alongside the CCS and the railhead, it had become his third parish.

That year Easter fell in the middle of the battle of Arras and reminded Bere that death was still the master in Flanders. By now he was overworked and exhausted, and when he muddled up the letters of two patients to their wives, the guilt stayed with him for weeks. Bere thought it was the intense, damp cold that had doubled the mortality rate at the CCS, with the surgeons he was so proud of not being given a chance to save the frozen men. The moribund ward – which Bere had renamed the Resurrection Ward – was busier than ever. There were days when they were admitting 300 new cases and all he had time for was to give Communion to the dying.

But day after day Bere went back to the wards, prepared to do whatever he could. One night when he was praying a man called him over. What did he want? the padre asked. I want you, the man replied, so Bere stayed with him for hours, simply holding his hand. When the man began to doze, the padre turned to the soldier in the next bed, who told him he was a chorister in his local church in Scarborough. They chatted softly about their favourite hymns and organ music, and finally Bere felt the grip on his hand loosen as the patient fell asleep. He waited a little longer to make sure the man was settled before leaving the ward.

It wasn't just the patients who needed him. Pressure on the CCS's staff had never been greater. He regularly visited the operating theatre with his soup-and-sandwich trolley. He did a weekly laundry round for them in town and collected their pay on his way back, so that when they returned to their tents at night they found clean clothes and money to send home. When the quartermaster injured his hand, he gave his wedding ring to Bere to look after, and the padre wore it for three weeks so that the man could see it was safe. To calm themselves in the evenings, the medics played bridge and, if there was no one to make up a four, Bere stepped in, no matter how tired he was – or how much he disapproved of gambling.

Finally spring came, the battle ended and Bere found time for his garden. An RFC station had been installed close to the No. 43, and several squadrons of aircraft and observation balloons took up residence. Bere was asked to give a weekly service, and in return one of the observers offered him a ride the next time it was safe to go up. So one sunny morning, when no guns could be heard, the doctors and nurses of the CCS stepped out of their tents and looked up into the clear blue sky to see their padre floating serenely above their heads, smiling and waving. But Bere wasn't just enjoying himself. Looking down onto the landscape below, he noticed an on old chalk quarry. He had been looking for chalk, because with the air base so close by, he was worried the CCS might become a target, so he wanted to paint medical crosses on the roofs of the wooden huts. As soon as the balloon had landed, Bere went off with a spade and a wheelbarrow to secure some chalk. The markings were duly made – and with the chalk left over he laid out a tennis court. He had been right to be worried. All through the summer of 1917, like everything else at the front, CCSs now became targets. At No. 11 near Bailleul a direct hit from a bomb killed four doctors and wounded five others. Twenty-three patients were killed and sixty-three were injured, as was the CCS chaplain.[23]

By August 1917 Bere was beginning to feel the strain. His world consisted of the CCS, the railway station and the POW camp, and time was marked only by the flowers he grew in his garden and the new graves that were dug in the ever-expanding cemeteries. The CCS was treating some of the worst cases he had seen; some of the facial injuries in particular were horrendous. The war, he concluded, was pointless. It seemed that nothing had been achieved apart from daily mutilation. The amputation ward was full and he spent several hours each week to prepare the men there for life back home. What sort of jobs might they find? One patient suggested they could form a troupe of circus acrobats. Bere laughed along with the others, but he worried about what awaited them at home.

At the beginning of 1918 there was talk again that this would be the last year of the war, but in the spring No. 43 was caught up in the swift German offensive and became the most forward medical post in the area. The numbers of wounded arriving were the largest since the Somme offensive. At Easter, Bere wrote home that he carried both his Bible and his prayer book, but had no time to open either. Patients arrived in great numbers, but he took pride in the fact that not one man passed the reception tent without bread and butter and a hot drink, unless he was unable to take it. Eating and drinking were not easy if your jaw was shot away, he wrote. In his work here during Holy Week he did almost literally 'wash his footsteps in the blood of the slain'.

Bere ran the reception tent every day for a week and then went to help out in the pre-operative ward. It wasn't usually until midnight that he and the other staff finally managed to get some dinner. There was the constant noise of shells landing nearby, but they were too hungry and tired to care. The enemy was almost within touching distance and Bere wondered what would happen if the CCS was captured. One padre had been running an aid post in an abandoned brewery. When it became clear that they would

soon be overrun by the enemy, he had calmly organised the full
evacuation of all patients and supplies. He and one of the bearers
had even given the place a quick sweep before they left, for a little
bit of swank.[24]

By mid-April the German offensive had stalled. For a while
quiet returned to No. 43, but Bere knew it wouldn't last when his
leave was cancelled. He had hoped to be at home for his daughter's birthday and take her to the zoo. Instead, he sat in his little
carpentry workshop and carved wooden crosses with tin name
plates for the graves that he knew he would be filling. Before long
the fighting started again and the padre used up every one of his
crosses. But when it stopped in the summer, even Bere started to
believe that the war was coming to an end. In the wards the men
were discussing who they would vote for in the election and how
they wanted to change the country when they got back. When
he went to the railway station, the trains were filled with POWs
instead of wounded. Yet the landscape he drove through with his
ambulance in search of supplies was a desert of shattered towns
and cratered earth. One day he found himself on a road going
through a cemetery – miles of desolation marked with little
wooden crosses. Sometimes he simply stopped the ambulance
and curled up on the floor in the back, trying to catch up on three
years of missed sleep.

When the Armistice came in November, everyone assumed
they would be sent home, but orders came that they were to stay
and look after accident and psychiatric cases. The mental wards
were given increased capacity and a specialist doctor arrived to
take charge of them. He sought out Bere and asked him to extend
his parish into the wards. Bere did his best with his patients, but
he was nervous of them. Their conditions were complicated and
he would need to learn more about them, otherwise he might
do more harm than good.[25] He continued his visits to the wounded
and the sickness wards and answered sackfuls of letters each week,
asking about the graves of loved ones. It looked as if he would
be in France for a good while yet. But then, during routine testing,

Bere was diagnosed as a diphtheria carrier. He was ordered to return home straight away.

Back in England, Bere only slowly adjusted to peacetime. He tried to explain to his parishioners what he had seen in France. He hadn't been in the trenches, he told them, but he had seen the war and all its suffering. As he tried to make sense – to himself and others – of his experiences at the Western Front, a new syllabus was being developed at the Army Chaplains Department training camp at Tidworth. It was a curriculum inspired by the work of chaplains such as Crosse, Doudney and Bere. Not only was the chaplain to be responsible for the spiritual welfare of the men, but he was also to look after their physical well-being and to show 'the spirit of help' in every way. The new padres were instructed how to find clean water and keep the men occupied. They were taught riding, cycling and cooking in a camp kitchen. They attended short courses on administering soldiers' pay, military form filling and the correct channels of communication within army bureaucracy. They learned map-reading and compass use, and in the medical classes they were taught basic first aid, how to apply field dressings and bandages, and the best ways of carrying the wounded.[26] The chaplain was to be the servant of his unit, the new syllabus stated, with a duty to serve everyone in every way.

Midnight on the battlefield of Loos, late September 1915.[27] A figure is suddenly silhouetted against flashes of shellfire in the dark. He bends to work, watched by men of both front lines straining to see what he is doing that can be so important that he risks a sniper's bullet or a stray shell. But for the man digging in the mud, there is no choice. He is burying the dead that lie all around him. He won't be able to get to all of them, but as long as he has breath in his body, as long as he can avoid the attention of the brigadier, as long as he can pull himself out of the deep trench every night and run and duck to find a way through the mire, then he will try.

There was heavy rain the night before. It made it difficult for the soldiers advancing across no-man's-land, but it made his job a little easier. If the ground is hard, he can barely manage two burials a night, but tonight the earth is soft, so he digs down into the wet soil until, quite quickly, a grave is made. Soldiers on both sides follow his movements, their eyes growing used to the darkness. They now realise what the man out there in the open is doing. There is absolute silence as he steps around a dark heap on the ground, which they know is a dead man. Lucky soldier, they think to themselves. Hope he gets to me, if I die out there. Not left to rot, but sent up to heaven by a good man and with a blessing.

They watch as the man carefully kneels down, trying to keep his balance. He bends over the body and there is a pause. They know he will be feeling around the neck of the dead man to remove the little round metal disc on its chain, ignoring the blood and worse that he might find there. He gently lifts first one hand and then the other, to see if there is a ring. He also checks in the man's pockets for a watch that he can return to his family. He sits back on his heels for a moment and fumbles with mud-clumped fingers at the buttons of his tunic pocket, to tuck away safely what he has found. Finally he bows his head, lifts his hands and speaks the words of the Committal. Then, rising from his knees, he rolls the man into the grave that he has dug and fills it again with the wet earth. Finally, taking one of the small wooden crosses tucked into his belt, he marks the grave. Then he moves to the next body. He works until dawn breaks, and when those who have been watching him on both sides get distracted by the line coming back to life in the early light, the man quietly disappears.

The soldiers of the 18th Battalion London Irish know who he is. Their chaplain, Father John Lane Fox, who has been with them on their journey from camp to battlefield, is helping the dead to rest.[28] Loos was a place of death, but their padre showed that even on the corpsefield there was room for love and the gift of service.

10

Ambulance Trains

Nurse Bickmore, Nurse Morgan,
Margaret Brander, Leonard Horner

The sensation of travelling as a parcel, put into the train and taken
out at appropriate times is very soothing.
Captain H. C. Meysey-Thompson, wounded at Bailleul,
21 September 1917[1]

Nurse Bickmore managed to lorry-hop all the way up to the front
entrance of the railway station specified in her orders. Here she
was to take up her new posting on board an ambulance train.
She had been assured that it would all be quite easy, if a bit
cramped: just turn up on time, get on board and check in with
Sister. Not much different from work at home. The ambulance
trains were like hospitals on wheels, carrying wounded soldiers
away from the battlefield to the base hospitals on the French coast
for long-term care – or, if they were lucky, all the way home to
England. The trains picked up the injured men from railheads as
close to the casualty clearing stations as could possibly be built.
Cables went out when a load of wounded needed collecting and
the nearest available train set off down the line. There were officers
on board and at the stations who were in charge of entraining
and detraining the wounded men. Bickmore had liked the sound
of an ambulance-train post. Like work at the CCSs, the trains
offered nurses the opportunity of real nursing. Having your own
carriage was like having your own ward. You had to keep it clean

and the patients were your responsibility, all the way to the end of the line.

When she went inside the station, it was dark and cold like a cave. It seemed completely deserted. She called out into the gloom, 'Hello, is anybody there?', but her words echoed round the vaulted ceilings and off the stone walls. No one replied. She wondered if it had all been a mistake. The whole station seemed to blur into one dark mass. Suddenly there was a quick flash of light, lasting just long enough for her to make out the closest train. This had to be *her* train, she decided. She started to walk towards where the light had come from, until she reached the end of the platform. To get to her train, she would have to jump down onto the tracks and walk over the tangle of rails and points – even though every good English child had been taught never ever to jump from a railway platform. She hesitated and wondered whether she had made the right decision after all. But she couldn't stand there for ever and there was no turning back now. She bent down low to put her hand on the edge of the platform and then lowered herself carefully onto the rails. She gathered up her cape and skirts and, grabbing her tiny valise, set out across the tracks. A number of times she almost fell, but she stumbled forward, the occasional glint of the metal rail alerting her to a new obstacle. Then she saw some small strips of light ahead of her and, as she focused on them, they solidified into a frame – it was a train window covered by a blackout blind. She continued to walk towards it, trying not to trip. Then, suddenly, there was a solid block of light as a door opened and a voice called her name, 'Nurse Bickmore?' A hand reached out to help her up a set of wooden steps.

Nurse Bickmore tried not to show quite how relieved she was by the sight of the soft, golden lights of the train carriages and the voice of the orderly who welcomed her on board. He took her valise and congratulated her on her light packing. Space was tight on board and some of these nurses packed as if they were going on holiday. Then he led her along the corridor to her sleeping quarters in an old first-class carriage. They had to stop constantly to stand aside and let people rush past carrying piles of linen and steaming kitchen pots. How could this entire world have been so well hidden in the dark cavern of the station? she wondered. But, more important, how would she ever be able to clear her uniform of the oil and soot stains from her journey across the tracks? The orderly apologised that she would have no time to rest, as the train was preparing to depart. Everyone else got to sleep at night-time, he grumbled, even at the front, but not the staff of the ambulance train. Night-time was for cleaning and restocking and getting ready for more patients. They had to sleep in shifts, whenever there was time. There wasn't time now, so when she had taken off her cape, she'd be reporting to the kitchen carriage to get a mop and some hot water.

As they left the sleeping carriage, the train lurched forward and Nurse Bickmore steadied herself with one hand on the carriage wall. You'll get used to it, said the orderly, and as she followed him along the corridor towards the kitchen car, the man warned her to keep her elbows in at all times. Then the train pulled out of the dark station and onto the open tracks, the wheels picked up speed and the carriage began to sway. She'd get used to that too.

Sister was waiting for her at the door of the kitchen carriage, steam misting up the windowpanes from the enormous vats of water boiling away on every gas ring. Nurse Bickmore was given a bucket of hot water and a mop and sent to her carriage, further up towards the engine. Get it ready, were her orders: sparkling clean, beds made, ready for patients arriving this morning. Keep the mop close to your body. Don't swish it about too much or people will trip over it. And keep an eye on the bucket: if the train stops suddenly, you don't want it tipping up and sending filthy water down the corridor.

Her carriage – her ward – was warm and bright from a row of electric lights along the wooden walls. It didn't seem too dirty. There were some brown stains on the floor that could have been dirt or blood, but they came off quickly. She only needed a couple of changes of water to get it all sparkling clean. Then she turned the lights down, as instructed, and opened all the windows to let the fresh air do its bit. The train was rattling along now in open country and the breeze was wonderful. She closed the windows again and began polishing up the brasses on the light fittings and doors. Next came the beds. Her carriage had four rows of triple-layer bunks, each with a sprung mattress. There was a pile of linen on each mattress – proper pillows and sheets and blankets. She hadn't expected to find such quality bedding. It took her a while to make up each bed, and the top bunk in particular was really tricky. She had to keep her balance on the ladder while reaching over into the far corner to tuck in the sheets and blankets. As she worked she realised there would be a lots of stretching and bending for her, once there was a wounded man lying up there, but he would be comfortable, in clean sheets, and that was what counted. Finally the carriage was done. Standing in the doorway, she looked at her work with satisfaction and pride.

As she walked back to the kitchen car to deposit her bucket, she paid attention to the contents of the other carriages. In some carriages there were seats for the walking wounded, cushioned and well built, like proper first-class carriage seats. In others she noticed frames and loops as well as seats: for stretchers, during pushloads, someone had told her. Pushloads – Nurse Bickmore noticed that whenever anyone said the word, their face froze for a moment.

By now it was light and the train was slowing alongside a platform. Bickmore took up her position by the carriage door, as instructed. She realised that she didn't know quite what to expect and was getting really nervous, so the sudden banging of the doors opening all along the train made her jump. Looking out of the window, she saw row upon row of bearers with stretchers lined up alongside the train, standing still, frozen like a ghost army. All of a sudden they started to move, pushing and shouting as they approached the train. Then the first bearer pushed past into her carriage, and soon stretcher after stretcher was loaded up in front of her. Even though she tried, she couldn't see much of her patients wrapped in their blankets, except for a glimpse of pale flesh. Bed by bed her carriage filled until there was no more space. The last bearer to leave caught her eye. All yours now, Nurse. Bickmore saw the exhaustion and strain on his face, his eyes bloodshot, unblinking. Then she was alone with her patients.

For the next hour Bickmore settled in the wounded men. She began by checking their tickets, trying to put names to faces. She noted those with a large red cross on their tickets: they were the most serious cases, and she would have to do everything for them. She reapplied bandages that had slipped, took temperatures and tried to pick up on any particular needs. One man had a bandaged jaw. Liquid diet, she noted, he'd need a straw: make sure to get one from the kitchen. She tucked in blankets and arranged pillows. She hopped up the ladders to the top bunks to make sure that all the men there had seen her face and knew she would care for them. Then the train lurched forward and they were off. Men cried out at the jerked movement. Bickmore flew between the bunks to find out what was hurting, then fetched more blankets and rolled them up to support fractured limbs.

When it was quiet again and they were rolling steadily, she went to the kitchen and fetched a huge vat of hot tea. In the carriage she handed it out in enamel mugs. It seemed that most of her patients finally started to relax. Bickmore stayed on her feet, walking the aisle between the bunks, watching, soothing, chatting and joking with the men. She handed out her first meal and afterwards, into the evening, her patients gradually began to fall asleep. She would have stayed on duty in her carriage for ever, but someone checked on her early the next morning and she was sent off to get some sleep.

After a week Bickmore had learned to pace herself, and much more besides. Tending her patients hour by hour, day by day, it felt the same as being on a hospital ward. Most journeys were so slow it was almost as if you weren't moving at all. Any ideas she had about trains steaming across France were soon dashed. A full train meant you could only travel at ten miles an hour, so journeys that would normally take hours often took days. Hospital trains occupied the lowest rung on the priority list for rail use, so they were always stopping to make way for other trains carrying troops, ammunition and supplies.

She also got to know the train itself. There was a dispensary in one carriage with up-to-date disinfecting apparatus for instruments. If patients could walk, they would be treated in dressing rooms manned by orderlies. Bickmore was most impressed by the store carriages next to the kitchen. As well as cupboards and shelving, they had huge barrels of water and ice chests. More water was stored in vats on the roof, although there could never be enough water for cooking, washing and cleaning. She also came to understand why British 'Khaki' trains were so preferable to French 'Green' trains. On Green trains there were no corridors, so staff in one carriage could only move into the next one by stepping outside onto the footplate and jumping across – how one was supposed to do this in a nurse's skirt while the train was moving was anyone's guess. The doors of Green trains were also very narrow, making it difficult to get stretchers up into the carriage. Moreover, Khaki trains had windows that could be removed to make way for bad stretcher cases and entraining under pressure.

After a couple of months Bickmore had become a train expert. She moved quickly and neatly along the corridors, elbows tucked in, always looking ahead for what was coming towards her. She learned how to change a dressing whatever the position of the patient and however cramped the space. She never wasted a drop of water. She could tell how full the train was just from the way it moved along the rails. Initially she enjoyed the speed of an empty train, but soon she came to associate it with what lay ahead – the grim, grey lines of bearers and the pale-faced men on stretchers – and she came to prefer the slowness and certainty of a loaded train heading for the hospital. She had learned to fall

asleep quickly and to wake suddenly; time on the train meant
something different from time in the outside world. She now also
knew what a pushload was, although she too never spoke of it
and couldn't bring herself to write about it to her family.

She learned not to mind the delays: hours sitting in sidings as
other trains flew past. Somehow time seemed less wasted if she
watched the view from the window with her patients, who were
speculating where the trains might be going and what battle they
were heading for. If they anticipated a long wait, staff even got
off the train – keeping one eye on the open carriage door – to
get some fresh air and stretch their legs or pick some flowers.
When all of a sudden the jolt came that meant they were off
again, the nurses would break for the train, scrambling up and
slamming the doors behind them, while their patients cheered
and cracked jokes about missing the 3.45 to Paddington.

Bickmore loved the joking in her carriage. She found that the
best jokes came from the men on the 'Blighty trains' heading
straight for the hospital ships to take them home to Britain. Blighty
patients had Blighty tickets and Blighty smiles. Blighty smiles were
the widest smiles of all and lasted the whole journey, however
long the delays, and by the end Bickmore found she was wearing
one too. But not all loads were Blighty ones. Some trains stopped
at the line of base hospitals up and down the French coast, and
the men knew they would be treated there and would probably
soon return to the front. Those loads were less cheerful, and she
had stopped counting how many times the men asked, 'Do you
think they'll send me home after all, Sister?' But at least they
knew they would be safe and looked after for a while.

When she went on leave for the first time she realised how
much she missed her train: it had become her home, and its crew
her family. While most people would spend the war cooped up,
she was permanently on the move, her feet hardly touching the
ground. She thought of the train almost as some living being,
warm and dependable, and knew its every noise and movement.
And she would never tire of cleaning her carriage. When she had

finished she would open its windows and let the night breeze renew them all.

Nurse Morgan, too, couldn't understand why anyone would want to work anywhere else. Her home was the No. 3 Ambulance Train. About 300 yards long and with a maximum capacity of 440 patients, it was a more basic model than Nurse Bickmore's train. It didn't have the luxury of built-in beds; instead it had iron stands and straps where cots or stretchers were hung. These made nursing difficult, because when the train was moving at speed the stretchers swayed and swung about. The nurses themselves had basic quarters with very little comfort or storage space. One day an enterprising orderly had come in with a carton of empty confectionery boxes that he had got from a French patisserie while on leave. He fastened the sturdier ones to the walls above each bunk to make little dressing tables for the nurses' mirrors and personal items.

Like all ambulance-train orderlies, those on board No. 3 were practical men. Not only could they repair the electrics and the gas supply, but when the cooks complained that the train's food-storage area was too small, they converted an empty carriage into a meat-safe by lining it with a wood-and-canvas frame with shelving, where the kitchen staff put trays of cold water to keep the temperature cool. So well did the storage work that No. 3 had fresh meat for its patients even in hot summers. Its kitchens produced good, hearty food – soups, stews, milk puddings – essential for malnourished men with nothing to look forward to on the long journeys but their next meal.

Something bothered Nurse Morgan as soon as she joined No. 3. There were no curtains on any of the carriage windows, so patients squinted in the glare of bright sunlight or were woken much too early in the summer. Others didn't like being stared at by civilians as the train slowed to go through stations. So she bought as much fabric as she could from a French haberdasher's and, in her free time, sewed curtains for every single carriage on the train, which the orderlies fastened up for her. A pair of curtains made each carriage a little more like a home. She soon looked for other ways to bring comfort to her patients. When the train stopped at a siding she always jumped down to pick flowers. One of her patients gave her an empty shell casing that he had polished up to a smart brassy shine, and it was never empty of flowers on a little shelf in her carriage. When word got round, Nurse Morgan soon had more shell casings than she could have imagined – and every carriage had a collection of highly polished vases full of French wild flowers.

The long hours on the rails or in the sidings gave everyone on the train plenty of time to get to know each other, and the patients always wanted to leave their nurses with a gift to remember them by. So Nurse Morgan didn't just get her artillery shells: she was also given road signs written in German, horseshoes and even a French roof tile, carefully saved in a kitbag and the only thing its finder had to offer the nurse who had eased his journey with such skill and care. Trains were generally chatty places, everyone talking all at once, carrying on conversations across the aisles. Nurse Morgan therefore paid particular attention to the men in the top bunks, who found it difficult to join in and could only stare at the wooden ceiling. She would spend hours up a stepladder, chatting to them and making sure that they were comfortable.[2] But she knew that not every train was full of happy men bound for Blighty with a shell casing in their kitbag. For each patient who was delivered home in soothing comfort, there was another for whom every jolt of the carriage was agony, the long journey a mixture of boredom and pain, and who cried themselves to sleep.[3]

It was in the summer of 1916 that Morgan felt she finally came to understand the war. They knew what was coming because they were delayed more than ever before; endless supply trains flew past them towards the front, and camps and depots sprang up overnight alongside the rails. Then there was no more time for flowers or presents, and the pushloads began to arrive. Unlike Nurse Bickmore, Morgan explained frankly to her family at home that a pushload was a train running at full capacity – no empty cots or seats, and all available back-up space used for stretchers. During the Somme offensive the pushload of 440 or more became the norm, as No. 3 struggled to keep up. Carefully planned entraining and detraining routines went to pieces in the face of the sheer numbers of casualties at the railheads, and within a week of the Somme the whole system of transit simply broke down.

Morgan realised just how bad things were when No. 3 train pulled into a base station to deliver its pushload, only to find 2,000 men who had arrived on an earlier train still waiting to be removed, with stretchers simply abandoned on the platform, the sidings and inside the station. There was not a spare inch of platform on which to detrain No. 3's patients, so the train sat there for hours until the previous arrivals were finally moved. Morgan tried to calm her patients, while all around them they could hear the moaning of men in agony, the train an island in a sea of human desolation.

But that was just the beginning. Soon afterwards they took another pushload to Le Havre and, as they pulled up to the platform, someone pointed out that all the other trains in the station were the dreaded TATs. Temporary Ambulance Trains were standard rolling stock pressed into emergency service and originally intended to move only the lightly wounded. Yet by the end of July 1916 they were being used to transport all sorts of casualties and arrived at their destination like a chain of charnel carriages; for the wounded men, the journey on these inadequate trains was agonising. As they watched the TAT wagons being unloaded at Le Havre station, a desperate medical officer asked the No. 3 staff for help with the detrained men. Nurse Morgan and a group of others volunteered to stay behind at the station after their train had left.

For almost two days they worked non-stop, constantly worrying that their supplies would run out and waiting for word that the base hospitals in town were finally ready to take in the wounded. But then they were told that the hospitals had no more room.

The train controllers were ordered to divert all trains from Le Havre as its station and hospitals were full to bursting point with casualties. Some of the nurses went out into the town to beg for supplies. Nurse Morgan worked on, trying to catch some sleep whenever she could, standing up or leaning against a pillar or a door, ten minutes here and there. Then, two days later, the base hospitals began to open again and their bearers came to take away the patients. When No. 3 returned to pick up its staff and Nurse Morgan felt again the movement of the train under her feet, she smiled with relief.

But the summer offensive went on and the pushloads continued. Whenever the train stopped at a railhead, more and more patients were loaded into every available space. There was also a new, unwritten rule: moribund patients were no longer taken on board. If their ticket said they wouldn't survive the journey, they were left behind at the railhead and the bearers would take them back to the CCS. As the train pulled away from the railhead, staff tried not to look back on the men who had been left to die.[4] Not that they had much time to think about it. At Vimy they picked up 436 patients, almost all having received no treatment except first aid from the bearers who had found them on the battlefield several days before. Often the men fell into a coma-like sleep as soon as they were laid down in the corridors or on a bed, and nothing could wake them. Their clothes and bandages were caked in mud and blood and it was almost impossible to keep the carriages clean. Sometimes all the nurses could do was shake out the blankets and then put them back on the patients.

Another time, 539 stretchers were somehow loaded onto the train, far in excess of its capacity. Stretchers hung from every strap and were laid out in the corridors, end to end. Morgan and the other nurses struggled just to move around the train, and their backs almost broke from the strain of nursing on their knees and trying to keep their balance. They toppled over onto their patients when the train lurched and gave up carrying vats of tea, as being too dangerous.

This was the hardest load she had to deal with. The wounded men's journey from the battlefield to the railhead where they were loaded onto No. 3 had taken two days. During that time they had received no medical care. There were spare uniforms on board, but before they could be distributed, and before any serious medical care could be given, each man had to be cut out of his uniform remnants and the mud and blood on his body washed away. With so many of them having multiple wounds, this process took almost a whole day; only then could treatment be given and new dressings applied. There was another reason why Morgan would always remember this load: it was the first to infect the train with lice. And it was when they found the bugs in their bed linen that the nurses finally lost patience with the whole damn war.

Only at times when a smaller load gave them some breathing space did Morgan have time to look out of the window and see what was happening in the outside world. She watched troop trains go by that were at least twice as long as No. 3, full to bursting with fresh soldiers for the front. Often she drew the curtains on her carriage so that the men couldn't see each other. At one station the train chugged slowly past an almost endless line of shells – so that's what they looked like before she turned them into vases. During another long stop in a siding they heard the cracking of anti-aircraft fire close by and climbed up onto the carriage roof to watch an aircraft weave and dive to escape before it was shot down. It was terrifically exciting, although no one knew whether it was friend or foe. It made Nurse Morgan take an interest in the war in the air. One of her patients on the next load turned out to be in the Balloon Observer Corps. He had fallen out of his balloon during a storm, but had got entangled in its ropes and only suffered some broken ribs, a broken ankle and some bad rope-burn. He drew pictures in her notebook of his accident and also showed her how to identify German and British aircraft.

In September the train was sent deep into the battle zone, further

nose, she realised that despite looking at the landscape of the war for two years, she had never stepped off the train to examine it up close. She found two other curious nurses and so they got their capes and gloves, jumped down from the carriage and went off to explore.

They soon became the centre of attention: the soldiers in the trenches thought the women were a kind of early Christmas present. Nurse Morgan found herself surrounded by men surreptitiously trying to comb their hair and get some of the mud off their faces. Someone at the back was even polishing his tunic buttons, and it was nice to see tunic buttons that didn't have a ticket tied to them. The men were keen to give the nurses a tour, and earnest discussions ensued about what they should see. Tanks first, no question. But could the nurses climb up and see the insides? Of course they could, Morgan thought. These were women who scampered over rail tracks in the dark and worked on moving trains. She loved the thought of being one of the first women in France to climb up and peer down inside the huge machines.

When they were walked over the frozen white battlefield, someone pointed out the German lines in the distance. Morgan had never seen the enemy so close, but it was an oddly empty experience. She could detect just a little movement here and there and some plumes of smoke. The Germans were just like them, she thought. Stuck at war over Christmas. Then the nurses were helped down a ladder into an actual trench, walking its length and seeing how the men there lived. They were shown a dugout and were impressed by its size and by the fire burning in the hollowed-out grate. Someone even made them cocoa, which was quite a treat: usually it was nurses making cocoa for the soldiers. Nurse Morgan returned to the trenches on Christmas Eve and Christmas Day, this time with almost all the other nurses from the train. It was then that she collected her very own shell casing, easing it carefully out of the ground after a soldier helped her find one that had gone off cleanly and wasn't too dented.

In return for their hospitality, she told the soldiers about her
work on the train. They were amazed to hear that only the driver
ever knew where the train was going, and that often they entrained
their patients without knowing where the railhead was or even
its name. They laughed when she told them how the train occasionally set off all of a sudden while they were still in the station
café or shopping in town. But there was no need to worry, she
assured the men. The train moved so slowly they could usually
catch up with it at the signal points.

When the time came for No. 3 to continue its journey, Nurse
Morgan stood on the footplate of her carriage to wave all the
soldiers thank you and goodbye. She hoped most sincerely not to
meet any of them again in one of her carriages, she told them.
As the train gathered speed, she watched the soldiers disappear
in the distance, grey coats against the snow, waving farewell. Then
the cold drove her back inside and the men went back to the
comfort of their braziers in the trenches – nurses and soldiers
returning to their different worlds of war.

Sister Margaret Brander started her service in France at the hospital
in Wimereux, where most of the Neuve Chapelle casualties had
been taken. When one of her best nurses died of cerebrospinal
fever, the loss drove her to ask for a transfer. She received orders
to report to the station on 18 May 1915 to join No. 10 Ambulance
Train. She would be the Khaki's senior nurse. When she turned
up at the station that morning in the pouring rain, the train waited
for her with a pushload of 265 patients. Sister Brander didn't even
have time to take off her coat before she found herself attending
to the wounded in their rain-sodden clothing and dressings.

It took hours to process them all – checking temperatures and
diet sheets, making sure they were fit to travel – and when they
had finished, Sister Brander went to sleep in her uniform, too
tired to undress. When she woke the next day they had arrived
at Rouen, where the men were detrained. The carriages were still
damp and humid from the rain-soaked men, so Sister Brander

ordered that all windows and doors be opened so that the train could be thoroughly aired before the next load arrived. After twenty-four hours on No. 10, it felt as if she had never worked anywhere else.

Yet it took some time to get used to being on a train. Although No. 10 was constantly moving, Sister Brander felt as vulnerable as she would have been at a casualty clearing station at the front. Collecting one load in the spring of 1916, the train was so close to the enemy guns that the carriages were shaking as the shells fell nearby. She hurried the bearers and chivvied the orderlies so that they could get going as quickly as possible. But it wasn't just the enemy she worried about. When they took in another push-load, there were so many men on board that their weight was too much for the train to bear and, with an awful-sounding crack and then a thump, the couplings snapped and the train slammed to a halt. Inside the overcrowded carriages men flew out of their bunks, landing on other patients lying on stretchers on the floor. In the kitchen carriage everything fell off the shelves and almost all the crockery and glassware was smashed; only the enamel tea mugs survived. It took the nurses hours to return the men to their beds, re-dress their wounds and calm them down. The kitchen staff and orderlies took almost as long to restore the kitchen and the stores carriages, and no meals could be served, only tea and water in the tough old mugs. Meanwhile the driver and his assistants rigged up a chain to reattach the carriages to the engine. It took three times longer than normal to get to base, and Sister Brander could feel the strain of the engine hauling their pushload, tearing and tugging along every yard of the track. Afterwards she was alert to every sound the train made: she knew that a sudden creak could signal disaster. The replacement crockery that she ordered was all made from enamel and tin.

Then there was the constant danger of derailment. The continuous traffic had worn out the tracks and throughout 1916 they were derailed several times. Although it wasn't particularly dangerous – the train was travelling too slowly to roll over or crash

– everybody was terrified by the sudden sensation of the carriages coming off the tracks.[5] Then they all had to get off, one by one, with the unconscious patients tied to their stretchers. They had to wait beside the train, sometimes in the rain or snow, and nurses and patients cheered on the orderlies who tried to lift the derailed carriages back onto the track.

Accidents further up the line, or a track damaged by enemy shells, could cause serious delays. Such delays not only put further strain on their tight supplies, especially the available water, but caused other significant disruptions as well. If the train was late returning to its base, it would miss the post or the payroll, which was bad for staff morale. It was often up to Sister Brander to fix things. As soon as they pulled into the base, she would run to the telegraph office to signal the army post service and pay-masters to reschedule their deliveries; and she became skilled at playing the sympathy card to get their attention. Often the supplies they were expecting had been loaded onto other trains, so the nurses had to buy what they could in town to restock their larder. An empty store carriage, concluded Sister Brander, was almost as much trouble as a carriage full of patients.

Despite all this, she came to love her train. After she paid a visit to a friend on another ambulance train she reported back to her team that it didn't come close to No. 10. She encouraged her nurses to pick flowers on their long stops and to keep the carriages bright and cheery. She was always concerned that the men got bored, so she spent much of her pay on books and magazines, which she distributed around the carriages. She loved the train year-round, even though each season brought its own problems. In spring her patients often arrived with their clothes drenched by the rain, and in summer the train would become insufferably hot. In autumn thick fog could slow the train to a crawling pace or stop their progress altogether. In winter it was difficult to keep the men warm, as the heating system only worked when the train was in motion and the engine generated steam, so when they had to stop the carriages soon became freezing cold. If they spent many days in below-freezing temperatures, their entire water supply froze; the orderlies had to light small fires underneath boilers and pipes to try and get it going again. One morning it was so cold that when a nurse started to mop the floor of her carriage, the water froze solid in minutes, turning it into an ice rink.

Each year Sister Brander was determined that they should celebrate Christmas, no matter where they were. Just before Christmas 1915 she wrote to her local newspaper describing her work, and in response she was sent enough donations to put together a small gift parcel for each patient, containing paper and pencil, a handkerchief, socks and a woollen scarf. They even had ham and eggs for breakfast on Christmas Day and plum pudding for lunch. Then one of the orderlies revealed that he had brought his bagpipes and he roamed the corridors all afternoon, the sound of his playing carrying from one end of the train to the other.

The train took Sister Brander to places, and showed her sights, she had never imagined. One night she woke when she felt the train slowing – always a bad sign. When she got up to find out what was happening, she saw a work party laying new track alongside theirs. They were working by torchlight and the scene had an almost fairytale quality, the men's silhouettes dancing in the flickering light. They encountered more and more work parties during the late spring and early summer of 1916, and she realised that a big offensive must be on its way. The groups of soldiers marching towards the front alongside the track got more and more numerous, and when the train slowly passed through one of the huge temporary camps, the noise of so many men in one place was unsettling for everyone. None of her patients slept until they were back on clear track.

One day, as they slowed to go through another camp near Abbeville, she noticed a soldier who was tied up to a post. What is this about? she asked her patients. Field Punishment Number One, Sister, said one. You get this for nothing, chimed in another. A bit of drinking, rowdiness, lip to an officer: you get tied to the post for an hour in the morning and an hour in the afternoon. Supposed to give you time to think about what you've done. But all it gives you is sunburn and not being able to itch your chats. By now the entire carriage was rumbling with resentment. Sister Brander was glad for the train to pick up speed and take her away from the senseless scene. Turning again to her patients, she smiled and talked brightly about something else – anything that would make them all forget the world beyond the window.

Leonard Horner joined No. 16 Ambulance Train in the summer of 1915. He was a Quaker – able to serve, but unable to fight – and had volunteered for the Friends' Ambulance Unit. Like everyone in the FAU, he had taken several courses in first aid and medical care in their Oxfordshire training camp before leaving for the Western Front. Initially Horner was pleased with his posting to No. 16. Everyone knew it was the best train in service. It had been privately commissioned by the United Kingdom Flour Millers' Association and consisted of fifteen of the most up-to-date coaches, with smart copper boilers, huge water-storage capacity and upholstered seating and bunks in carriages painted a bright white.[6] But within days Horner began to lose his enthusiasm. To start with, the train was difficult to clean. It had 708 windows and Horner grew to hate every one of them. In addition, the smart white paint showed every speck of dirt and got chipped every day, so after every inch of it had been washed clean, he had to touch up the paint with a brush. Having spent his first day on the train cleaning, Horner wrote to his family that evening requesting several sets of overalls so that his smart FAU uniform wouldn't get stained.

Then there were the large water tanks. When he was shown them on his first day, no one mentioned how they got filled up. At some railheads there was overhead water storage with pipes and pumps, but most of the time they had to be filled by hand.[7] Any train staff who could be spared dismounted and formed a line from the tanks to the mains supply, passing buckets along one after the other. The line often stretched across the entire railyard, over platforms and into goods sheds, where there might be only a single tap to fill one bucket at a time. It took hours to fill up the tanks. Sometimes, at smaller railyards, locals would join in the line to help them and then it wasn't so bad.

Throughout the autumn of 1915 there were very few casualties aboard No. 16 and Horner got bored. And although the carriages were empty, he was still cleaning them, day after day. When one evening another orderly pointed to the unpicked bunches of purple grapes that were withering on the vine in the French countryside, Horner felt that he too was going to waste. The next day he requested a transfer to a despatch-rider unit. While his request was being processed, his letters home got more and more angry about the injustices and privations of life on the train.

He hated the delays most. They spent so much time just waiting to move on, with nothing to keep them busy except more cleaning. When there was fog they couldn't see any debris or damaged tracks ahead of them, so derailments were common. Horner almost broke his back the first time he got out with the others to try and lift a carriage back onto the rails. When fog was thickest, the train moved as slowly as it could and one of the orderlies walked ahead, looking out and alerting the driver to any obstacles. At other times the fifteen carriages were too heavy for one engine to pull them up a steep hill, so additional engines had to be sent for. This meant more delays and, as Horner soon found, delays begat delays. No. 16 had been specially designed to take patients right up alongside the hospital ships waiting in port, and the train ran to the ship timetable, which was driven by the tides. So if they were delayed, they missed their ship and had to wait at least twenty-four hours for the next one, to the dreadful disappointment of their patients, who thought they were on the last leg home.

Yet worse than delays was damage to the train – and it wasn't always caused by the enemy. In a tunnel outside Rouen they passed a heavy goods train whose load had come loose and it scraped along one side of No. 16, breaking every single window-pane, ripping off all the door handles and leaving deep scratches in the carriage walls. The repairs took over a week and the train's staff had to find and pay for rooms in Rouen while they waited. But damage from enemy fire was more common. Trains became easy targets for German guns. The engine's smokestack was visible from afar in cold, clear weather, and increasingly aircraft were sent out especially to look for trains. One such air raid landed no direct hits, but still smashed 250 of No. 16's windows. Another destroyed the kitchen carriage, so there was no food or hot water: staff and patients had to make do with cold drinks, bread and biscuits. They had to pull into the nearest railhead, which was located next to an ammunition dump, and while the mechanics worked hard to repair the damage, no one slept that night for fear of another air strike. With the shells nearby, they knew that this time they were likely to be blown to pieces. Although the repairs weren't finished, they decided to move on the next morning.

When the train entered the battle zone, it often came under fire. Once they were shelled during entrainment, and orderlies and bearers had to dive under the carriages, leaving the poor patients on stretchers to their fate. A Quaker brother from another ambulance train told Horner that one time they were pulling away from a railhead with a pushload when the enemy broke through the lines close by and a huge number of British soldiers suddenly appeared alongside the slow-moving train. They jumped on, desperately hanging on to footplates and couplings as the train got them all away to safety.

But then, sometime in 1916, Horner withdrew his request for a transfer. He had to acknowledge that he had begun to enjoy being on his train. He had got used to its rhythms and quirks, and the strains and groans of the engine no longer irritated him. Instead, he found himself urging it on under his breath as he worked: Come on, old boy, you can make it. His family knew that his mood had changed when they received a letter asking for tins of toffee for his patients. One night the train stopped in open country and Horner climbed out on the roof to look at the stars. He could see the whole night sky and tried to pick out the constellations he had learned at school. In his next letter home he asked for star charts.

Each ambulance train was a community on wheels and Horner now tried his best to improve morale among the staff. He helped put together a newsletter, as recommended by Quaker HQ for all ambulance trains, featuring plenty of jokes as well as reports on flora, fauna and the astronomy visible from the train roof.[8] He organised a chess tournament, carefully timed so that the finals took place in the last hours before arriving in port. There was also a football team and, when the train stopped at a casualty clearing station for more than a day, the train's orderlies would arrange a match against its staff; Horner looked the other way when some of his patients placed bets on the outcome.

No. 16's staff constantly had to adapt to new situations. In the autumn of 1917 more and more patients arrived on board with infectious diseases in addition to their wounds. Horner suggested that they allocate a quarantine carriage to prevent staff and other patients from getting infected with meningitis, flu or rheumatic fever. Ambulance-train staff were more likely to fall ill than any other units at the front: a train was simply too confined a space ever to be completely cleared of bugs and viruses. Horner also organised the supplementary carriages that were needed to care for a load of mental cases, who had to be kept in confinement. These were attached to the end of the train and had their own staff. One night one of the patients escaped by jumping out of a window. As he was suffering from religious mania, Horner tried to get him to return by calling out religious exhortations into the darkness, but they were unable to catch him. The fugitive was later found in a prison for deserters in Rouen, and the train's medical officer who collected him assured the staff there that he was not a coward, but delusional.

Horner was also put in charge of the carriages for POWs that were sometimes attached to ambulance trains to transport them to camps. This was work he really enjoyed. It was interesting to meet the enemy up close, and they didn't seem all that different from his own side. Most of all, they were a good source of souvenirs. Horner swapped cigarettes and French currency for the best war trophies – Luger bullets, woollen uniform caps, crests, badges, even a time-fuse from a German bomb – which he sent back home to his family. But despite his pleadings and his offers of many boxes of cigarettes, he was never able to get the most valuable trophy of all: a German helmet.

One day, when Horner looked out of the window and saw a despatch rider going by on his motorcycle, he felt a sense of relief that his transfer hadn't come through. Not for him the lonely life of mud-spattered goggles, rutted roads and shouted orders. He worked on the smartest and best-kept ambulance train. He was part of the closest community serving at the Western Front. By the end of the war, No. 16 train had carried over 150,000 passengers from the front to the ships for Blighty. Quaker histories noted what Horner already knew: that the Friends' work on the train was the most consistent and solidly useful done anywhere at the war.

II

Furnes Railway Station

Sarah MacNaughtan

I have an interesting job now, and it is my own, which is rather
a mercy.

Sarah MacNaughtan, 5 December 1914

Late one evening at No. 1 Belgian Field Hospital an ambulance
driver wandering the corridors found Sarah MacNaughtan
restocking a linen cupboard. They were short-handed, he explained
to the nurse. They needed someone to help them unload the
ambulances at the railway station at Furnes, where the patients
would be put on a hospital train. There wouldn't be much for
her to do: just a bit of help with the lifting, sorting out personal
belongings, linen and such. A spare pair of hands. Everyone knew
that Miss MacNaughtan never said no; usually she didn't even
need to be asked. She was older than most of the staff at No. 1
Belgian Field. She was also a wealthy, intelligent and sensible
woman, and when she saw a problem she wanted to solve it. So
she got her coat and hat and climbed into the cab of the ambulance.

It was a short journey into town, but she was tired and had to
force herself to listen to the chatter of the driver. They were
observing the blackout in town and she couldn't tell one building
from another as they drove carefully through the streets to the
station. They could barely see to unload their patients, but they
got them down and MacNaughtan walked ahead to find a place

for the stretchers. It was even darker inside the station than outside and it took a while for her eyes to get used to it. She had expected an empty platform, with a few porters and bearers waiting about with torches, having a quick smoke, ready to take their patients from them. Instead she seemed to have stepped into a nightmare. The whole platform was filled with wounded men lying on stretchers, blankets or just a bit of straw. She couldn't see any porters or bearers – simply a blurred mass of broken men, abandoned in the dark.

Somebody waved at her. Did she know when the train was coming? She shook her head and picked her way carefully back towards the station entrance. They couldn't leave their patients here; they'd have to take them back to the hospital until the station was clear. There's no point, said the driver, it was like this most nights. Hospital trains were always late, and sometimes they were delayed by whole days. Her guess was as good as anyone's as to when it would arrive tonight. And no, there were no staff to look after the injured in the meantime.

MacNaughtan went back into the station and wandered as far along the platform as she could, picking her way through men and stretchers. There were patients from her own hospital, men she had nursed just days before, who she had thought would be safely in Calais by now. There were groups of men from other hospitals further away. Worst of all, there were men who had come here straight from the battlefield, wearing the bloodstained dressings applied at the aid posts and with the mud of the trenches still coating their uniforms. When the men heard the rustle of her skirts as she walked past in the dark, they asked her for water, chocolate or a bit of bread, as they hadn't eaten since the day before. A sudden thought stopped her in her tracks. She realised why no one was looking after the men: no one knew they were here. They had been forgotten in the darkness and cold, everybody thinking they were someone else's responsibility.

Nurse MacNaughtan took off her hat and coat, rolled them into a bundle and went back to the waiting ambulance. She told the driver to return to the hospital. She and the bearers would be staying. She would need the ambulance's torches and medical supplies; in fact, she'd need everything in the ambulance that wasn't nailed down. Waving away his questions, she told him to send someone to collect them at sunrise. The bearers looked at each other, but didn't argue. You didn't cross Miss MacNaughtan when she had that look on her face.

MacNaughtan had noticed a goods shed to one side of the main hall. It would do for an instant medical post. After clearing it, she laid out the supplies from the ambulance. It wasn't much, but they were used to doing a lot with very little at No. 1 Belgian Field. She asked the bearers to patrol the hall with their torches and bring her the very worst cases. Soon the goods shed began to fill with stretchers. MacNaughtan knelt on the cold, hard floor and treated the wounded with the few supplies she had. She cut dressings into the smallest usable pieces, and removed those hurriedly applied on the battlefield. She tore bandages into strips, and gently supported broken limbs. She found a small sink in one of the station corridors and began to wash away the worst mud and blood that caked many of the wounds. The water was cold, but at least there *was* water. She found a tin mug from somewhere so that the thirsty men could have a drink.

She worked on for hours, until 3 a.m., her eyes red and strained, her back and joints aching. She had treated everyone the bearers had brought her, but there were still so many men outside on the platform. She simply didn't know what else she could do for them. Then one of the bearers stuck his head round the door: he had heard the hospital train in the distance. Soon smoke, light and the noise of train doors banging open against carriage sides filled the station. MacNaughtan stood motionless as one by one her patients were carried off. None of the train staff seemed to notice her presence. She had done too little, she thought. She had redressed a few wounds and applied some splints, but the men on the platform had been hungry, thirsty and cold throughout the night. Tomorrow would be different.

At sunrise the ambulance came back for her and the bearers. In her room at the hospital she saw the deep bruising on her knees, caused by hours of kneeling on the hard shed floor. Every joint burned and she could barely move her hands. But it wasn't pain that kept her awake that morning: it was the knowledge that more work waited for her at the station. By midday she was up, writing a list of things she needed. Then she went to the market in Furnes to buy coffee, bread and vegetables. From the hospital kitchen she got two huge marmites and portable stoves, and as many enamel mugs as the staff were willing to give her. From the medical stores she took dressings, bandages, splints, blankets and morphine. Bearers loaded it all into an ambulance and then she returned to Furnes station. There she found a fleet of ambulances, their bearers unloading wounded men and carrying them into the station, with more arriving from every direction.

The stationmaster was surprised that one of the ambulances brought supplies and a determined English nurse. MacNaughtan assured him that she wouldn't be a burden on him and his staff. All she needed was an empty corridor with a sink and a hook for her gas lamp. Station staff and bearers unloaded her ambulance, bringing in the supplies as the station platform grew crowded once again with wounded men waiting for the next hospital train. Then the staff left, wishing her luck and silently thankful that someone was taking charge. MacNaughtan immediately fired up the burners on her stoves to prepare coffee, cocoa and vegetable soup. Some of the men from the previous night had gone, but the hospital train hadn't been able to take them all. They were soon indistinguishable from the new arrivals. By the light of her single lamp she saw hands reaching out for a mug from her tray. It was all right, she kept repeating. There was plenty for everyone – she'd be back with more.

And so began Nurse MacNaughtan's second night at Furnes station. She filled and refilled hundreds of cups and tended the badly wounded; she changed dressings and handed out half a morphine tablet here and there along with the cocoa and the soup. Gradually the station seemed to come to life. Men sat up and warmed their hands on their mugs. Those who had the energy exchanged a few words; there was even some laughter. When the hospital train finally arrived at the first light of dawn, its bearers and orderlies were surprised at the transformation. There was none of the silence and heavy cold they remembered from previous journeys. Instead the patients seemed lighter, and the staff could smell coffee, not blood. This time the station was emptied completely, and when the wounded men had all gone, MacNaughtan began to wash up hundreds of tin cups and scrub the cauldrons so that she was ready for the next night.

From then on, caring for the abandoned men on the platform of Furnes station became Nurse MacNaughtan's sole purpose. She thought of little else, running between the markets, the hospital and the passage that became her kitchen at the station. On that first evening she had taken over an eight-foot stretch of corridor, but by the end of the first week the entire corridor was hers, and instead of one gas lamp on a hook there was now a whole string of them. Four stoves burned under the cauldrons and there were sacks of onions, potatoes, leeks and cabbages, together with bags of dried peas and lentils and boxes of coffee, cocoa and sugar – all paid for out of her own pocket. Other staff at No. 1 Belgian Field gave up their precious spare time to help her. By the second week the improvised kitchen was full of nurses sitting on vegetable sacks, laughing and chatting as they peeled and chopped ingredients for the soup, while orderlies filled baskets with chunks of bread. The station came back to life, just like some of the men lying on the platforms, who lifted themselves up and tried to comb their hair tidy whenever a nurse approached.

MacNaughtan and her team soon outgrew the corridor, so the stationmaster found her a proper room. It had an electric light, shelving and cupboards, so at last she could organise things properly. More and more nurses and orderlies joined her, and there were now three cooks working on the stoves during the busiest periods. She no longer had to worry about supplies, either: the town's shopkeepers dropped off their sacks of unsold vegetables at the station every evening. Within the military hierarchy there was relief and gratitude for MacNaughtan's work, conveniently expressed in a lack of interference.

She thought constantly about how to improve things. Making use of her own wealth, she ordered a little wheeled trolley with a hot plate from Harrods, which made the soup distribution much easier. When she noticed that many of her patients came in with cracked and broken boots, or with no shoes at all, her next order was for 1,000 pairs of the thickest wool socks that Harrods sold. Each evening, after the first rounds of drinks had been served, she loaded up her trolley with the socks and gave them out to anyone in need. One French officer lifted himself up to take a pair, but then suddenly turned his head away. As she moved closer, she saw that he had only one eye and it was full of tears. Was he all right? she asked. Did he need medical attention? Were the socks suitable? 'Madam,' the man replied, gathering himself and attempting a small bow, 'in these socks I could take Constantinople.'

But MacNaughtan had a secret: she herself was chronically ill. She suffered from a form of anaemia that was incurable and that affected her joints and her circulation. So when she returned each evening to her room at No. 1 Belgian Field, she tried not to look at the bruises on her arms and knees, which never seemed to heal. Under her uniform her legs and arms were as thin as sticks, except for her joints, which swelled and burned when she sat down for too long. She was never able to sleep much and although she was handing out food all night, she almost forgot about eating herself. Only the hospital chaplain noticed her frailty and did his best to comfort her. He waited up each night and, when she returned from Furnes station, he helped her down from the ambulance. He always managed to save a plate of food for her, kept warm somehow, and sat with her in the kitchen while she ate. If there was no food left or she wouldn't eat, he found a bottle of port from somewhere and poured her a good glass. The chaplain was also waiting for her when she returned from the station on Christmas Day. She had worked alone, as most nurses and orderlies were on leave, and she returned midway through the bitterly cold afternoon, staggering up the stairs of the hospital frozen and exhausted. When she summoned the last bit of energy to get into bed she found a warm hot-water bottle there, organised by the chaplain.

It wasn't just MacNaughtan's physical health that was frail. When she first arrived in Belgium, it had all seemed so simple: she had come to save lives and nothing else mattered. But as the war was grinding on, producing more and more casualties who were waiting helplessly at Furnes station, it was harder and harder to keep going. She had found it easier in the early days, when it was just her and the two bearers in her improvised kitchen at the station. Now that she led an entire team, she found it difficult to stay cheerful all the time and motivate the others. Her religious faith was also beginning to crumble under the strain. She knew that there were so many similar railway stations across the front, where men lay quiet and bleeding in the darkness and where there was nobody to care for them. One early morning when she returned from the station, a regiment of Belgian soldiers passed her on their way back to the trenches. They wore patched uniforms, but their little band played a jolly tune. She waved to them as they marched past and, when they were gone, she burst into tears.

Some of the casualties she encountered at the station revealed the worst of the war. There were men with horrific facial injuries, stripped of their dignity and their ability to speak. She saw how they watched the other men eat and drink. Only a few had somebody to help them feed through a straw. Most were beyond help and would soon die. One evening she looked across the station to see a mental case struggling against the bearers who tried to hold him still on his stretcher. Although he twisted and strained he didn't make a sound; there was no raving and screaming, but total silence. She had to remind herself that this wasn't a dream. She was awake and at Furnes station.

At the end of 1915, after more than a year in Belgium, Nurse MacNaughtan returned to England. Her doctors prescribed rest, but instead she gave talks about her work and raised money for war bonds before returning briefly to the war, working as a nurse in Russia. She was in London waiting for a new posting when her health collapsed in the spring of 1916. Sarah MacNaughtan died at her home in Mayfair in July at the age of fifty-two.

Shortly before she died she had written:

> Some people enjoy this war. I think it is far the worst time . . . I have ever spent. Perhaps, I have seen more suffering than most people . . . I see them by the hundred passing before me in an endless train all day. I can make none of them feel really better. I feed them and they pass on.
>
> One reviews one's life as one departs. Always I shall remember Furnes as a place of wet streets and long dark evenings with gales blowing and as a place where I have always been alone.

12

Wounded

Joseph Pickard, Moreuil, Easter Sunday 1918

Came back to England with a pyjama, monkey jacket and one sock.

Joseph Pickard, 1986[1]

Joseph Pickard joined up in 1916, claiming that he was as old as the century. It was a lie. He was just fifteen, but in the Year of Battles no one at the local recruitment office bothered to check such details. Pickard wanted the war to make a man of him, although by anyone's reckoning he was as adult as they came. He had started work at the age of thirteen in a large factory making fishing rods, Hardy's of Alnwick. Made out of Tonkin bamboo, Hardy's rods were the best in the world. It was delicate and demanding work, so Pickard was no child when it came to attention to detail and dedication. But when he arrived in France, someone saw that he looked awfully young, so he was assigned to a bearer team at a field ambulance behind the lines until he was old enough to fight.

This wasn't what Pickard had in mind. He wanted to be part of the action, not clearing up afterwards when it was all over. Things improved only slightly when the bearer team was temporarily assigned to move shells. The Flying Pig mortar bomb weighed sixty pounds and had a sensitive fuse, so it couldn't just be lumped about from one place to another, but had to be moved by men familiar with the transportation of heavy but delicate loads. Pickard's team were so good at it that they were soon sought

after by the artillery companies. They used to move two Flying
Pigs at once, strung up on a pole between them. Pickard was
keen to stay with the artillery men to watch them fire the shell
he'd just lugged over the jagged landscape, but he was always
chivvied away. It was like being back at school.

Pickard hated his job as a stretcher bearer. His hands always
hurt, more than they had ever done at the factory, and when he
returned from one of his carries and set the stretcher down outside
the CCS, the nurses and doctors wrongly assumed that the blood
on his hands was the casualty's. One night the pain was so bad
that he cried himself to sleep. There hadn't been time to get his
hands treated at the medical post and the next day he would have
to do it all over again. He began to worry about his job prospects
after the war: there would be no job for him at Hardy's if his
hands were mangled.

That day he had spent almost all his time carrying a seventeen-
stone officer, and his palms and fingers were cut to pieces. But it
wasn't just the man's weight that had angered Pickard. Officers,
he had decided, were the worst kind of carry. On another occasion his team had picked up an officer who demanded to be
brought back to the rear on the most direct route – not for him
the long-winding but safe journey through the trenches that had
been carefully worked out by the bearers. If they made the whole
carry on top they were likely to get shot at, but the officer said
it was an order. The best the bearers could do was tell him they'd
have to wait until after dark. So they sat there and waited for
nightfall. No one spoke. Surely the officer must realise now that
he had made a mistake. Finally the lead bearer said it was safe to
go and they set out. Pickard was getting angrier and angrier with
every step of their carry. His rage did not go unnoticed and the
officer threatened to report him. But Pickard refused to be intimi-
dated. He thought that the officer's injury was so light it looked
suspiciously like a self-inflicted wound. He was getting good at
spotting those, and he let the man see that he was suspicious. In
the end the officer didn't report him.

Yet even more annoying than pig-headed, cowardly officers were carries that didn't stop crying and whining. Some of them were moaning like babies, while others were shouting for their mothers. It didn't do them any good, except attract snipers and get them all killed. Quite often Pickard told them to shut up. The bearers were doing their bloody best, and if the wounded didn't shut up, they'd leave them there out in the open and they could try to find their own way back.

When he got too frustrated with his bearing duties, the team leader sent him back to the Northumberlands' camp so that he could calm down. The war was turning into a huge disappointment for Pickard. Most of the time he was bored or hungry. Being hungry was worse than being bored. He was a growing lad and needed his food, but the rations were never enough. And if they were under fire, the men delivering the rations just left them by the side of the road and yelled at the soldiers to come and collect them. Worst of all, he thought he would never see any action. Every time he was sent back to the Northumberlands, they were either pulled back or there wasn't much going on in their part of the line. This wasn't what Pickard had been looking for.

But then the war found him. Easter Sunday 1918 was the day when Joseph Pickard grew up. At Moreuil, the Northumberlands were defending their lines against the enemy incursions that were part of the great German spring offensive. Pickard was as far forward as possible, firing as the enemy approached the British trenches. They were coming much too quickly, he thought as he loaded and reloaded. Then something hit him, as solid as a sandbag, knocking him off his feet, and he lost consciousness. When he woke up he couldn't work out exactly what had happened. He was alive, but he was hurting, and he was in a trench full of corpses.

Pickard knew he couldn't stay where he was. If the advancing enemy found him he would be killed by a bullet or a bayonet. But as he tried to stand up, his legs gave way and he crumpled back into the mud of the trench. So he stayed down, wrestling his little first-aid kit out of his pocket and trying to work out where he had been wounded. His hands and arms seemed to be fine, so he felt carefully all around his body. He found that he had been hit three times – in the leg, in the back and in the face. He wasn't sure exactly what the damage was to his back and face, but he could feel enough torn flesh and splintered bones to know that it was bad. He put the only field dressing he had on his leg and wrapped the gauze bandage around it, while blood from his shattered face dripped down onto his hands. Then he sat down to gather himself, trying to ignore the growing pain in his back and stomach. Crawling seemed the only practical thing to do, so he dragged himself out of the trench and set off over the muddy ground, the enemy guns sounding all too close behind.

He was able to raise his head, despite the pain and the blood running down his face into his mouth, and when he saw khaki uniforms ahead he called out. Three men came running towards him, one of them a friend he had made from among the Northumberlands. When they bent down to haul him up, he saw the look of horror on their faces. He must look a bloody mess, he thought. They loaded him onto a stretcher they had found, as gently as they could, and set off. Pickard tried not to cry. He tried to be the good patient that he wanted his carries to be, but it was hard. His friend saw his pain and comforted him, trying not to look too hard at the hole in his face. There was also blood coming from Pickard's stomach now. They were lucky that an ambulance drew up alongside the little party and told them to put him on board. The three soldiers waved Pickard away with a mixture of relief and sorrow. They were certain this was the last they would see of the prickly teenager, who was hungry all the time and talked mostly about fishing rods.

Pickard was achingly thirsty, but the ambulance driver had seen his stomach wound and wouldn't give him water. As they drove on, he passed out again. The ambulance pulled up at a dressing station that seemed hopelessly overrun with casualties. When he was unloaded and examined, he woke up long enough to hear the staff talk about his wounds. The shrapnel in his back had sliced through his sciatic nerve and exited through his bladder at the front, smashing his pelvis along the way. No wonder he hadn't managed to get up; it was a miracle that he had been able to crawl. His leg was all but shredded and his nose had been blown clean off. He heard the harassed doctor say that he had no doubt this was Pickard's last night on earth.

The doctor told the bearer to place his stretcher in the moribund area of the dressing station and alerted the chaplain that there was a man in need. In quiet tones the padre administered the last rites, with the doctor standing respectfully by. Pickard was dimly aware of the chaplain's voice through the fog of agony. Then the doctor gently placed the blanket over his head and left him to let nature take its course. When his friend arrived at the station and asked after him, the doctor shook his head. There was no hope. Could the friend help with the paperwork, so that his family would be informed quickly? Pickard's name and details were noted and a field postcard filled out to be sent to his mother. Then they started to dig his grave.

But Pickard refused to die. Sometime later that night a nurse noticed the blanket that covered his face rising and falling as he struggled for breath. She immediately told the doctors and a team of medics rushed over, pulling back the blanket. Mumbling apologies, they began to clean and dress his wounds. They gave him some water through a straw – Pickard would always remember it as the sweetest medicine he had ever tasted. They knew they had to get him to a hospital as quickly as they could, and there was an ambulance leaving in a few minutes for the hospital train. Because officially he was dead, he had no ticket to tie to his tunic. But anybody who saw his wounds would know that he was Blighty-bound, no question.

The journey was a new kind of hell for Pickard. Now he finally understood why his carries cried so much. As he was borne from aid post to cart and from cart to train, every jolt of the stretcher sent flashes of pain down his leg, up his spine and through his stomach. Being loaded onto the train was even worse, though they put him in through a window rather than bumping him up the stairs of the carriage. His perforated bladder failed him over and over again, and he sobbed as much in apology as from pain. The nurse who saw him to the top bunk of the three-berth Khaki train placed a small ladder against Pickard's bed so that she could climb up and check on him.

The train crawled towards the port, stopping every hour to let troop and supply trains pass. The movements of the train caused him further agony. The nurse spent long periods perched on the ladder, holding Pickard's hand. He had been given all the morphine tablets he was allowed, and perhaps a few more, but the drug seemed to make little difference. When he had the energy, Pickard reached up and placed his palms flat against the slatted wooden ceiling of the carriage, trying to steady himself against the jerks and surges of the train. But it didn't make much difference. He was only semi-conscious when he was taken off the train. He passed out completely on board the hospital ship.

When Pickard reached London and was put into the care of the London Ambulance Column he had further deteriorated and was no longer able to speak. Arriving at Victoria Station, his lack of ticket meant that he wasn't on anyone's hospital list, so nobody knew what to do with him. Almost an hour passed on the platform while this was debated, but then a nurse who had space in her ambulance agreed to take him to a hospital. No one was expecting him there, either, but eventually a doctor admitted him and filled in the required paperwork. It meant that Pickard was officially alive again.

Pickard always maintained that his mother had second sight. When she received the telegram advising her of his death, she simply refused to believe it was true. Yet it was several weeks before she received confirmation that she was right. She told his friends in town and at Hardy's what hospital he was in, and many of them went down to London to visit him. It took Pickard a long time to recover and, when he finally went home, people stared at his broken face. But he didn't mind it much. He had gone to the war to become a man, and a man he now was, even if he didn't look or walk quite right. One day a child asked him what had happened to his nose. He had lost it in France, he replied, and there wasn't any point in going back and trying to look for it.

13

The London Ambulance Column

Claire Tisdall

And so I find myself back in one or other of London's stations in the dim light of the semi-blackout. The air is heavy with soot from the old steam engines and fetid with the smell of stale poison gas and gangrenous wounds.

Claire Tisdall, 1976

In the evening of 11 November 1918 Nurse Claire Tisdall wrapped herself in her big blue cape and got ready for duty as usual. When she got on a bus she hoped it would take her all the way to Victoria Station, but as she got closer to central London, every street teemed with excited people, singing and cheering the end of the war. Eventually it became obvious that the bus wasn't going anywhere through the crowds, so she got off and continued her journey on foot. She heard people around her talking about the future – what life would be like, now the war was finally over. She tried to imagine her future, but couldn't yet see beyond the work waiting for her on the platforms of Victoria Station. She suddenly began to feel fearful and decided to think about the past rather than the future. And she needed to hurry, otherwise Mrs Dent would be angry with her.

The thought of Mrs Dent took her back to her very first day with the London Ambulance Column when she had met her on the doorstep of a large Georgian house in Regent's Park in 1915.[1] Tisdall had never been inside such a big and elegant building and now she was being chivvied up the stairs to the registration office. All around her people were coming and going, pushing and shoving, carrying beds and desks and filing cabinets, shouting at her to get out of the way. She squeezed past a group of men moving a wardrobe down the stairs and eventually found the office. She was given a form to fill out and, while she waited, she looked out of the window. The driveway was filling up with ambulances and vans bringing more supplies. It was almost as if the Dents were expecting the Germans to invade Regent's Park.

The brisk and busy nurse seated at the desk brought her back to reality. Did she know what the London Ambulance Column was? Tisdall admitted that she didn't. The friend who had told her they were looking for volunteers said they needed nurses working nights, so there would be no disruption to her daytime job. Did Tisdall remember the first casualties coming back from Ypres at Christmas last year? It had been chaos. Nothing had been ready for them, but worst of all, there had been no transport to get them to the hospitals. There were trains to bring the wounded from the coast, and hospital beds ready to receive them, but no real thought had been given to how they got from one to the other. Hospitals only had a small handful of ambulances, and there was no one to care for and supervise the men who got off the trains. The wounded soldiers were left for hours in the dark and cold, while a few drivers and orderlies struggled to cope.

The nurse paused to check that Tisdall understood, before continuing. The London Ambulance Column had been formed, with official approval from the Red Cross and War Office, to bridge the gap. It was paid for almost entirely by Mr and Mrs Dent, whose family had made a fortune in Hong Kong and who had also donated the huge house. The column had its own fleet of ambulances, its own staff and its own supply chain. Those vehicles she could see out of the window were part of a fleet of 140, each with a driver. In addition, the LAC would have fifty nurses and a corps of bearers and orderlies. Employees of Derry & Toms formed the first group of volunteers, and the department store had also donated all the linen that Tisdall had seen being delivered. Young Mr Toms himself was leading a group of bearers. Upstairs there were twenty-five telephone operators and administrators who waited for calls from the Red Cross telling them when the hospital trains were expected. The trains would always arrive in the evening, after the commuters had gone home. The operators contacted the volunteer nurses and orderlies and, if they didn't have a phone, sent a despatch rider with a motorcycle. Then they would all be off to the stations to collect the men. The column loaded the wounded into ambulances and saw them safely into hospital, making sure that they were comfortable along the way. No injured man would ever be left by himself on a London platform again – not if the column could help it.

For Claire Tisdall this was exactly what she had been looking for. As a single working woman she had tried to find a way to contribute to the war effort, but she couldn't knit, and sitting in a town hall rolling bandages didn't seem enough. She'd even attended a few nursing courses, but there seemed no way to use her knowledge alongside her work. She couldn't lose her job: it was her salary, and her brother's army pay, that was keeping the family out of poverty. She had been forced to give up her dream of reading English at university, and she now sat night after night in their shabby home, listening to her parents endlessly lamenting their state. No, working evenings and some late nights would not present a problem for her.

The nurse signed Tisdall up immediately, discreetly checking for an engagement ring. Nothing. A single girl meant fewer distractions. Then she sent her to collect her uniform: a long white skirt, a linen cap and a thick, navy-blue woollen cloak. They were already being called the Bluebottles, said the supply manager. Over the next few weeks Tisdall completed the training programme, quickly working her way onto the more advanced courses. Mrs Dent herself took the last class. She wasn't going to give them more medical talk, for there were better-qualified people in the column to do that, but what she had to say was equally important. They must, above all, learn self-control. They were going to see things at the stations that would make lesser women faint. But they weren't lesser women; they were the LAC, and they would at all times be quiet, unobtrusive and polite. There would be no fainting, no panicking. The schedule would be kept to and the ambulances would leave on time. The wounded men and the men yet to be wounded would be relying on them and, if they couldn't cope, the Red Cross would have no hesitation in closing them down. She wished them good luck. She would see them all at the station when the next call came.

A few days later Tisdall was sitting at her desk when the company telephonist put through a call from Column HQ. Tisdall was required at Waterloo Station. She had been told to keep her uniform at work, so she went off to the staff lavatories to change. She stopped for a few seconds to look at her new self in the mirror: Nurse Tisdall would be making her contribution to the war effort that night. Her colleagues sent her off with scattered applause and widespread admiration and she caught the bus to the station. On the platform she met her fellow nurses, lined up parade-style as they had been trained. Mrs Dent came over and handed her a typed sheet. Tisdall had been allocated three patients, all stretcher cases. She had to find her ambulance and her driver and take the wounded men to a large general hospital in Kingston. Tisdall tried to memorise the information on the sheet, but when a train whistle sounded in the distance, she folded the paper and put it in her pocket.

With a long screeching of brakes and clouds of steam, the train engines ground to a halt along the platforms. Then the doors banged open and the train orderlies jumped out, followed by the bearers. They began to call out the names of each hospital and Tisdall listened hard until she heard her destination. She ran over and introduced herself, but the orderly wasn't listening. Instead he began to recite the state of her patients: whether they were conscious or not, needed a dressing change or a drink, and if they were likely to die en route to the hospital. Tisdall tried to take it all in, but she was distracted by the exhaustion visible on the orderly's face and by the blood on his tunic. She also noticed an odd, deathly smell that hung about him.

When she stepped inside the carriage she saw that it had no seats or luggage racks. Instead stretchers hung from the ceiling or were stacked in bunk frames. Wounded men waved at her weakly, hoping she was coming for them. Mrs Dent had called for unobtrusive politeness, so she calmly walked along the rows, nodding and smiling and checking tickets until she found her men. She introduced herself and told them that she would be accompanying them to hospital. Then she stood back to let her bearers hoist them down and out of the carriage. When they were heading for the station exit, she paused to look back at the scene inside. The station was full of trains and there were so many carriages like hers, full of so many men undone by the war. She gathered her cape around her and caught up with the bearers to lead them to the ambulance.

One of her patients was bleeding under his dressing, so she thought it was better to put him on the bottom rack of the ambulance to prevent his blood dripping on the men lying underneath. Then she double-checked her supplies and sent the bearers back. Now she was alone with her patients. Was everyone ready? She folded down the little wooden seat in between the stretcher racks. Then they were off. The streets of London were empty, so the driver sped smoothly towards the hospital. She watched her patients to see whether the ambulance's movement was causing them pain, but they seemed quiet enough. One of them even managed to sleep. At the hospital a team of bearers was waiting for her. They unloaded the wounded men and she explained their conditions as briskly as the orderly had done earlier. The driver offered to drop her off near her home. He had to go back to Regent's Park anyway, to dispose of the bloody linen and get the ambulance ready for the next run.

When Tisdall turned the corner into the street where she lived, she could see in the moonlight how dirty her uniform was. There was blood on the apron and cuffs and soot on the skirt. It would all need laundering. But she had passed the test: she had done what was expected of her. She noticed that she was breathing calmly for the first time in hours. Then, standing outside her front door, she began to cry. Slowly she composed herself, found her key and opened the door. Trying not to wake her parents, she quietly went upstairs to her room.

That was the only time she cried during her time with the London Ambulance Column. But it wasn't that the work got easier or that she got used to it. There was no getting used it, not when you saw the broken men coming off those trains, but she felt that if she started to cry again, she might never stop. Instead she somehow learned to detach herself from it, so that she could get on with her work. When she later looked back on her first night, she couldn't even remember why she had cried. It had been an easy night. Only three patients and one trip to Kingston. She would soon learn what a pushload was: that it meant carriages crammed to the rafters with wounded men, some flung straight onto the train from the battlefield and having received little medical care in the meantime. Some nights she thought she could smell the contents of the trains before the doors opened. Often she worked all night, from the dark of the semi-blackout to first light, loading and unloading the ambulance, speeding back through the city streets, rushing to get to the men still waiting on the platforms. Back at work the next morning she prayed that no call would come that afternoon so that she could get some sleep through the night.

But there was never enough rest. Exhaustion became the natural state of column staff. If there weren't enough bearers to be found, Tisdall had to help carry her patients. Victoria wasn't too bad, but Waterloo Station had sets of metal stairs that you had to go up and down to get out to street level, so sometimes she had to lift the stretcher right above her head to keep it level. Then she had to struggle through the melee of other nurses and bearers with their patients, all calling for their drivers. Sometimes they also had to unload the patients themselves at the hospital, if there was a heavy intake. They had to find their way around a strange building, trying to locate a doctor or nurse, and then retrieve their blankets and pillows after the patients were delivered. And all the while they knew there were other men still waiting for them on the station platforms.

By Christmas 1915 column work had become Tisdall's world. When she later looked back on the war, she couldn't remember any details of her day job, just the nights when the ambulance was speeding through the dark and quiet city. And while outside everything was dim and silent, inside the station there were squealing brakes and escaping steam, there were men shouting and crying. It was a world that had its own smell, of soot and rot. And it was a world where long hours of waiting were followed by shorts periods of frantic activity. The trains brought the front right into the heart of London, the tracks a poison trail that led all the way back to France.

While they were waiting the volunteer nurses had each other for company, but after long hours in the cold even chatting became tiring. Often they were starving. If they had been summoned straight from the office, they didn't have time for supper, so usually there was a whip round for change for the chocolate machines inside the station. Finding drinking water was also difficult, as station managers usually locked the lavatories at night. And in winter they were cold. The ambulances weren't warm at the best of times and there were never enough blankets. To stay warm Tisdall stocked up on hot-water bottles from the column stores and, as soon as the trains arrived, she ran to the locomotives to ask the stokers to fill them up for her. After a while she knew how to find the right valve and fill them up herself, waving her thank-you to the driver.

There was some real excitement on nights when the paper boys arrived with next day's newspapers. Then the volunteer nurses would stand together and read the latest news of the war. Getting the fresh print ink all over their hands and uniforms, they would speculate about which battle had produced that night's casualties. The columns were as well informed as anyone in the country about the war, but it wasn't just the headlines they got first. They were the first to see men who had been gassed, with the smell of the gas still clinging to their woollen uniforms, greatcoats and the blankets they had been given at the aid posts. Often it mixed with the stench of gangrene, which poisoned the men's flesh. No matter how long the orderlies had left the train windows open on the ride from the coast, the patients arriving in those carriages would be dopey and slow to transport.

From July 1916 there were gassed soldiers in every single push-load that pulled up in the London stations. The first time Tisdall entered a carriage full of gas casualties, she fainted and had to be revived on the platform. Apologising and getting back on her feet, she took a deep breath and went back inside. Gas cases made their lives more difficult. They had damaged lungs and needed to sit up for the whole of their journey to hospital. Nurses had to be alert to the slightest change in their breathing. Tisdall found it easiest to sit on the floor between her gassed patients so that she could focus on them above the noise of the ambulance engine.

Later Tisdall couldn't remember a time when she entered the station and didn't smell gas. When it was really bad, all the flowers bought by well-wishers to welcome wounded men turned black and died. But then flowers had no practical use at the stations, she thought. Cigarettes, on the other hand, were always welcome. There was nothing more that a wounded man returning to Britain wanted than a bath, a bed and a smoke. The Dents arranged for hundreds of packets to be delivered straight to the station. Tisdall always remembered to take plenty of matches and made sure they were kept dry. She later wondered how many cigarettes she had lit since 1915 – thousands probably. Even patients suffering from burns, whose heads were swathed in bandages, wanted a smoke, and she had to learn how to put a cigarette in their mouths through the dressings and light it so that she didn't set fire to the gauze. Bring cigarettes, she always told people who asked what they could do to help, not flowers. But they brought flowers anyway, and they drooped and died in the station's gas-polluted air.

By 1916 the public were coming to the stations in increasing numbers. On sunny summer evenings a large crowd gathered outside whenever word got out that a train was due. They would cheer every ambulance that passed them heading for the hospitals. At first, Tisdall had been alarmed by the large numbers of people, but she soon saw that the reception heartened her patients. She opened the canvas flaps at the back of the ambulance and helped the men sit up so that they could wave. And if it was a warm evening, she tied the flaps back and pointed out the landmarks of the capital as they drove past.

By the end of 1916 Tisdall was beginning to wonder whether she would ever feel rested again. After a night on duty, she went straight to work in the morning and there were too few nights when she was able to catch up on her sleep. She had no social life and her family had started to complain that the only time they saw her was when she was asleep in the parlour armchair, too tired even to go upstairs to her room. But for Tisdall the column had become her family. The volunteers didn't know much about each other, often only their surnames, but they knew what the others went through and what they were capable of. There were two middle-aged ladies who regularly invited everyone back to their house for hot stew or soup at the end of the night. Those nights round their kitchen table were the best of all, warm and sustaining. Tisdall also made friends among those working at Regent's Park. Everyone knew 'Despatch', as they called the messenger with his various motorcycles, leather gloves and goggles, who criss-crossed London to gather the volunteers. Then there was the youngest volunteer of all, only a schoolgirl by Tisdall's reckoning, who had begged her parents to let her nurse in France. They had refused, but allowed her to join the column, so every evening she arrived at Regent's Park, took up a post in the corner of one of the supply rooms and put pillow cases on pillows, hundreds of them, night after night. Tisdall always tried to give her encouragement and tell her how grateful they all were for her work. Each ambulance was supposed to have a complement of blankets and pillows in fresh white cases, and when the patients saw them they felt they had already arrived at hospital. So by helping to make them comfortable the schoolgirl was a nurse after all, Tisdall told her. The girl beamed at the praise and added another pillow to the pile waiting for the ambulance drivers.

In 1917 trains started to arrive with special carriages for POWs. Tisdall could speak German, so she was always allocated these patients. One night a young German officer cried continually in the back of her ambulance. He kept pointing to his leg and, when Tisdall examined it, she found that he had ruptured his femoral artery. She applied pressure, as she had been trained, and managed to keep him alive until they arrived at the hospital. For months afterwards she was teased by the other volunteers about getting a letter from the Kaiser. It was strange to think that the first life she had actively saved was that of a German soldier, but a life was a life.

Not all the carriages arriving at the London terminals brought wounded men for the column to deal with. Some trains had unmarked grey carriages, right at the end, which stayed locked while the column unloaded the rest of the train. Tisdall had thought that they were supply carriages, but one night she saw orderlies she didn't know start to open the doors and release footplates. And, later on, when her driver took a shortcut away from the station, she saw a small fleet of grey ambulances, also unmarked, parked down a side-alley. Eventually she discovered from one of her bearers that these carriages and ambulances were for mental cases. No one, not even the experienced volunteers of the column, were allowed to see them. Tisdall would never again ask any questions about the grey transport. Her ambulance once carried a badly shell-shocked, wounded chaplain. All the way to hospital he shivered and trembled, and he wept constantly. Tisdall was astonished that one man could produce so many tears. Then the sobbing suddenly stopped and the man was still – he had died of fright. If the men in the grey carriages were likely to be in a worse condition than the poor padre, then Tisdall didn't want to know.

As 1917 went on, the loads became heavier. The column staff now got special leave from their employers, and many volunteers slept at Regent's Park on camp beds during the day. At Easter, Tisdall worked seventeen nights in a row, with only brief naps in between. Then one night off, before returning to the station for twelve more nights. By now every train was a pushload, every carriage seething with gas and blood. But it wasn't just the nurses who were suffering under the strain. The column's drivers spent hours crossing the capital, their eyes straining to see the way ahead on the dimly lit streets. It was all too easy for them to fall asleep and lose control of the vehicle. One really foggy night, Tisdall's driver began to nod and then fell asleep at the wheel. The ambulance suddenly jerked to one side and mounted the pavement. Tisdall fell off her little seat, bumping her head on a stretcher frame. The patients were thrown out of their stretchers and screamed in agony, their stitches ripped, their broken bones unset. Tisdall calmed them and returned them to their stretchers, patching up their opened wounds as best she could. As the ambulance continued its journey to the hospital, she could hear the mortified driver sobbing in his cab.

The year 1917 took its toll on everyone. Mr Dent had a breakdown and retired from column work. Mrs Dent carried on, but the volunteers began to feel beleaguered, as if they alone in all of London were fighting this war. The city seemed oblivious to their sacrifice, as every night the telephones rang and telegrams summoned them to yet more work. Sometimes they begrudged the lights behind the windowpanes as they drove through the capital: as the city ate and slept, they tried to soothe a desperate man in the damp darkness of the ambulance. Their employers became less understanding of their absences and their exhaustion. Tisdall often sat at her desk unable to concentrate, and her colleagues tried their best to cover for her.

It didn't help morale that the public's attitude was beginning to change. The crowds still came to the station, but sometimes it was to gawp at the horrifyingly wounded men in the ambulances. At the New End Hospital in Hampstead, when ambulances had to slow down to turn into the driveway, people would try to catch a glimpse of the men in the back. Tisdall tied the canvas flaps tightly, but somebody would lift them up and call out what he saw there to the others.

By the beginning of 1918, Tisdall knew she was close to breaking point. But every time the call came, she still took down her navy cape, wrapped it around herself like armour and went out into the dark. And every so often, just when she thought she couldn't cope any longer, something happened that revived her spirits. Once her ambulance was stuck in traffic and she heard the call of a flower seller nearby. She dug around for a few coins in her leather purse and jumped out of the ambulance. She told the driver not to worry – she was just going to buy a bunch of violets. When the flower seller saw her running towards him, he told her to put away her purse and pressed the whole tray into her hands.[2] At that moment the traffic started to move again, so she jumped back into the ambulance, calling out her thanks. She folded down her little seat and sat with the tray of violets on her lap for the rest of the journey, breathing in the scent and freshness that filled the whole ambulance.

Then there was the time she had spent all night going back and forth between the station and a hospital in Richmond with some of the worst cases she had ever seen. Several of her patients had died en route. At dawn Tisdall was alone in the back of the ambulance with piles of bloody dressings and the empty stretchers stacked on the floor. The driver told her that he would take a shortcut through Richmond Park as the gates had just opened. When Tisdall leaned forward to open the canvas flaps, she suddenly smelled grass and could see the bright-green leaves of the trees in the old Tudor hunting ground. The sun was shining and it was going to be a beautiful day. Dew glinted in the distance, the last of the daffodils moved their heads in the breeze and the park's deer looked up, unconcerned, as they passed. A soft wind blew away the smell in the ambulance and Tisdall almost cried at the sudden beauty of it all. Whenever she thought of the war, its poison and ravages, she also thought of that morning in Richmond and the peace it had given her.

Now it was the last day of the war and, if she could think of Richmond, maybe she could believe that peace had finally arrived. A final push through the crowds and Tisdall arrived at Victoria Station. An orderly was waiting and hurried her through, closing the door behind her. As soon as she was inside she saw that, in here, the war was far from over. There was the steam and the poison, the shouts of the bearers and the clanging of the trains instantly drowning out the elation in the streets. The procession of stretchers leaving the platforms had already begun. And suddenly anger and misery gripped Tisdall's heart, harder than ever before. The war was not over; it would never be over, she thought. Somewhere in her mind there would always be the soot and gas-poisoned air of the station and of the war.

That night Tisdall and her driver made the slowest journey across town in three years of column work. They were going to a hospital in North London and had to cross the centre of town. They could not avoid going through Trafalgar Square. By now there were hundreds of thousands of people gathered in central London and they had been singing and flag-waving and cheering to the point of hysteria. Every street was clogged and, as much as the driver tried, weaving in and out of side streets, he could not find a clear way through. No more cheering for the ambulances, Tisdall thought. It was as if they had become invisible, the crowds – with their flags and joyful faces – preferring not to see them.

When the driver leaned out of his window asking people to move, they took no notice and simply sang louder. The ambulance was now crawling forward at a snail's pace. It was difficult to see what was in front of them, and many of the faces that pressed against the windows were red and glassy-eyed from drink. Tisdall tied down the canvas flaps tightly so that her patients wouldn't be frightened, but the vehicle was jostled and bumped from side to side as the crowd pushed against it. She had to hold the stretchers in their racks steady so that they wouldn't be dislodged as the ambulance rocked on its thin tyres. In Trafalgar Square on the last day of the war, in the middle of the ecstatic celebrations of peace, Tisdall and her patients cowered in the dark of the ambulance, in mute fear, praying the driver would get them through.

They finally made it to the Regent's Park ring road and picked up speed. Tisdall held the hands of each of her patients in turn, trying to offer comfort, but they were all numb, confounded by the journey. Outside the hospital too there were crowds dancing on the pavements. No one seemed to notice them as they pulled into the driveway and the hospital staff came out to collect their patients. Suddenly Tisdall felt terribly lonely, and for the journey back to Column HQ in Regent's Park she climbed into the cab and sat beside the driver. They unloaded the dirty linen and dressings together, and Tisdall took it up to Laundry whilst the driver swept out the back. He was still there when she came back out and she waved goodbye. She passed Despatch going into the building and was going to call him, but then faltered. In four years of working together she had only ever called him Despatch: she didn't know what his real name was. She promised herself that she would find out before her work with the column ended. It would be her resolution for the first day of peace. Then she wrapped her navy cape around her once again and began the long walk home.

Epilogue

No one survived the Great War unscathed. The wounded had their scars, as did the men and women who cared for them – although theirs were less easy to see. The country as a whole had been wounded. The war was like a lesion on the collective brain of the nation. The lesion was a cruel condition; there was no memory loss; instead, there was too much memory – for the soldiers of their wartime experience, for the families of the loved ones they had lost. Everyone had lost someone – husband, brother or son, neighbour, workmate or pal. But it wasn't just the dead who were mourned. Many of those who made it home were lost too, pale shadows of their former selves, unable to explain what they had suffered to families who would never be able to understand.

A few days after his wounding, **Mickey Chater** wrote home to his family: 'Well my dears, I had such a charming birthday charging German trenches that I am now in hospital.' It took a year in hospital in France before he was ready to come home. His injuries were so complex that doctors had almost given up on him, but his life was saved when one of the pioneers of facial surgery took over his case. Charles Valadier was particularly proud of the work he had done to reconstruct the young soldier and wrote about it in a medical journal, giving Chater a copy just before he left his hospital. Chater married his girlfriend, Joy, at the end of 1916 and they had a son. But the Mickey who came back was a shadow of the Mickey who had marched away, head held high with dreams of glory. He was more serious and everyone noticed his fragility. Despite his injuries, he tried to return to France, but it was clear that he would never again be a soldier, so he worked for the Ministry of Munitions until the end of the war. In 1919 he joined the family paper business, from which he retired in 1967.[1] When, after his retirement, he was asked by the Harrow School Old Boys to give a lecture on his war experiences, it wasn't quite the speech they had expected from someone who had participated in the battle of Neuve Chapelle.[2] Much of it was taken up with his gratitude to the medical staff who had worked so hard to save his life in France. When Chater died in 1974, Valadier's journal article was found carefully preserved among his papers.[3]

It took **Bert Payne** almost two years before he was ready to leave hospital. He didn't take to the enforced inactivity and was soon up and about within the hospital walls, volunteering to work as an orderly. His doctors were as grateful for his resourcefulness as his COs had been in France and put him to work in the VD ward, to spare the female nurses. Despite being in considerable pain and on a restricted diet because of his injuries, he became one of the most senior orderlies in the hospital, relied upon to draw up diet sheets, distribute medications and assist the radiographer. His girlfried, Joey, had waited for him and they married in May 1918. When Armistice was declared, Payne took almost no notice. He was determined to get on with his life and not even the unveiling of a Pals' Memorial in Montauban meant very much to him. Yet like Chater, he would never quite recover. The physical damage to his face was obvious and his jaw didn't work all that well, so Joey learned to make soft food that he could chew. But there was other damage, less immediately obvious. The returning scout was a harder man than the one who had gone to war. He became less forgiving of weakness and intolerant of failure, especially by members of his own family. Most of all, he despised all wars. 'War is ridiculous,' he once said. 'You can't win. You kill a lot of men and they kill a lot of you and when you've got there, you're there in any case.' His children were a little afraid of him, but his grandchildren found him fascinating. He painted them pictures of the phoney tree he had discovered and they were never quite sure whether or not the story was true. Then they went to the Imperial War Museum and saw from their display that it was. Bert Payne died in 1982.[4]

Joseph Pickard endured years of operations before finally being released from hospital in 1922. When he went home to Alnwick, there were no jobs for him at Hardy's, as he had feared. Instead he found work at the Birtley Instructional Factory, set up after the war to provide jobs for soldiers, where he trained as a watch-maker. The damage he had suffered to his back meant that he was in pain for the rest of his life, but he was unable to secure a decent disability pension from the Army. Joseph Pickard retired in 1959 but lived on in poverty until his death in 1988.

John Glubb was the exception. He never lost his physical scars, but he would always relish his part in the Great War. It took a year to put his face back together. One of the surgeons was William Kelsey Fry who, unable to return to France because of his own injuries, was now operating on soldiers at the Army's new facial hospital at Sidcup. Glubb knew of Kelsey Fry's war record and was honoured to meet him. During a month's recu-peration he took a voluntary job to stave off boredom when he was harangued as a shirker by a housewife. He demanded that the surgeons finish repairing his face as quickly as possible, so he could return to the front. He didn't need his old face, he said, just a face that worked. By the summer of 1918, a year after his wounding on the Menin Road, the surgeons had finished with Glubb. It didn't look pretty, they warned him; his strong boxer's jaw and chin were gone for ever. But he didn't need to be pretty where he was going and the Army didn't care about his lopsided face. They needed seasoned officers more than ever to counter the last enemy offensive.

When the war ended, Glubb was determined to go on soldiering. In 1920 he volunteered for duty in Mesopotamia and fell in love with the Arab world. He single-handedly raised a camel corps of

Bedouin tribesmen, leading them to a series of victories, and when the kingdom of Transjordan was created as part of the post-war settlement, he resigned his commission and was made principal military officer to King Abdullah I. His Bedouin corps became the Arab Legion and for decades it was the most formidable military force in the region. In 1956 Glubb retired with the rank of lieutenant general and returned to Britain, where he wrote a series of popular memoirs of both the Great War and his time in the Middle East. He was knighted the same year. Glubb was the last man ever to be given the title of Pasha, but he was just as proud of the name given to him by his Bedouin troops: Abu Hunaik, or Father of the Little Jaw.

Few stretcher bearers wrote about their experiences and very few at home understood what they had been called upon to do. **Earnest Douglas, William Young** and **William Easton** were all decorated for their courage during the Year of Battles, but all three were captured during the last Great German offensives of 1918. Nothing is known of Douglas and Young after their return to England, but Easton volunteered to remain in Germany, where he worked in a POW camp hospital after the Armistice. There he was desperately needed: after the German defeat, the staff, including all the doctors, had simply left the camp and gone home. Easton nursed the remaining patients in the hospital until they were all strong enough to return to Britain in 1919; he was demobbed the following year. Struggling to find a job, he realised that his medical experience was of real value and applied for a position in a hospital for amputees in Bristol, where he worked until his retirement.

Regimental Medical Officers had all had medical careers in civilian life before the war, so many of them simply resumed it when they came home.[5] **John Linnell** was one of those, but **Geoffrey Hardwick** decided to put his experience to good use and continued his work in the RAMC in the Mesopotamia campaign. His family believes he would have stayed in the RAMC but he returned to Cornwall in 1926 to take up general practice inherited after the death of his father. He was a GP and local Medical Officer of Health for Newquay. He always had a particular interest in dermatology and his family understood this to come from the war years where he dealt every day with skin conditions such as trench foot, trench fever (caused by the bite of a body louse), lice infestations and rat bites. He died relatively early, at the age of 64 from cancer. There is no word of whether the ferrets were ever able to make the adjustment to peacetime ratting. Both Linnell and Hardwick were decorated for their service in France.

William Kelsey Fry never returned to the front, but he remained one of the war's most popular and remarkable RMOs. When he had recovered from his injuries the RAMC decided to draw on his dental surgical experience and sent him to a new hospital at Sidcup, set up specially for facial casualties and run by the surgeon Harold Gillies. It was the perfect posting. Kelsey Fry had the quiet confidence to inspire staff and patients in an untested hospital doing innovative work. Gillies could be difficult, but remembered that 'Captain Kelsey Fry turned up for duty . . . and put us in his pocket straight away.'[6] Everyone at Sidcup soon became fond of him, even Henry Tonks, the notoriously grumpy artist who kept the hospital's diagrammatic records and who gave Kelsey Fry two pictures that he painted of work in the operating theatre.[7] After the war, Kelsey Fry took up a post at Guy's in the Dental School, but as soon as war broke out again in 1939 he volunteered for service. Once again he would find himself at the cutting edge of casualty treatment. He was sent to East Grinstead, where he designed and built the reconstructive dental unit for Archibald McIndoe, which after the war became the leading centre for postgraduate study in dental surgery. In 1951 Kelsey Fry was knighted and he continued his work, writing the key textbooks on his specialism, until his death in 1963. An old comrade from the Fusiliers, writing to *The Times*, made the following contribution to his obituary:

He was steadfastly courageous, devoted to his battalion and to his task. His calm and happy temperament carried him unstrained

throughout all that long period. He was immensely kind . . .
Needless to say, the battalion loved him, and particularly that little
band of outstanding stretcher bearers whom he inspired and with
whose survivors he remained in touch. That is the man we
remember with gratitude. Other good men followed him, none
quite reached his stature.[8]

Anyone visiting Kelsey Fry's home remembered two things
about him above all others: his smile, which never dimmed, and
the greenhouse where he grew his beloved carnations. He always
wore one in his buttonhole. His photograph, complete with smile
and carnation, was used by King's College London in their student
recruitment material for the academic year 2010–11.

Surgeon **John Hayward** returned home to Liverpool and retired
soon afterwards. **Norman Pritchard** came back to a civilian career
at King's College Hospital. **Henry Souttar** remained at the Army's
hospital at Netley until the end of the war and retained his interest
in physics.[9] He even married the daughter of a physics professor
and wrote several textbooks on the application of physics to surgery,
as well as designing equipment for Netley's recuperative physio-
therapy departments. He never forgot his time with Marie Curie
at No. 1 Belgian Field and was an enthusiastic pioneer of radium
therapy. His post-war work was as influential as his achievement at
Furnes. In 1929 he wrote and illustrated *The Art of Surgery*, which
remained the standard textbook for decades, and throughout his
career he designed and built surgical instruments. He was knighted
in 1949 and died in 1964, at the age of eighty-eight.

Jentie Patterson left No. 3 CCS when her father became seriously ill and her sister Martha could no longer nurse him on her
own. She returned briefly to France, first as a nurse on a hospital
ship and then, in March 1916, to ready an entirely new CCS, No.
16, for the coming offensive. No. 16 was one of the most up-to-date
CCSs at the front. The living quarters were excellent and there was
even a bath hut. But when her father's condition was declared
mortal Patterson went back to Scotland and nursed him until he

died. The records of the Royal College of Nursing indicate that she continued to nurse after the war and never married. **Winifred Kenyon** left nursing soon after the war, presumably to get married, but saved all her mementos of her time at the CCS, including the newsletters that reported the results of the Hare and Hound races and the fancy-dress competitions. Nothing is known of Nurse **Elizabeth Boon** except for the letter she wrote to the family of Private Simpson in Tottenham after his death. The letter, and the care and devotion it showed, meant so much to the soldier's family that they donated it as a single item to the archives of the Imperial War Museum. Private Joseph Simpson is buried in the Terlincthun British Military Cemetery in Wimille, plot number X.E.4.

Both orderlies, **Alfred Arnold** and **Harold Foakes**, survived the war and came home. We know almost nothing about their lives afterwards, except that both men married and had families, who one day sat them down and made them write up their memories of the war. It was a similar story for the hospital-train staff. **Nurses Bickmore** and **Morgan** got off their trains in 1918 and nothing more is known of them, except the few memories they jotted down of their time in France. **Margaret Brander**, like Jentie Patterson, went home and contined nursing for the rest of her life at the Perth Royal Infirmary. Her will established a scholarship in her name to support student nurses of limited means. Quaker **Leonard Horner** was demobbed in 1919 and formed the Old Sixteeners' Association, so that the close friendships made on the rails of France would not be lost. One of their first acts was to bind up the train newsletters into hardback volumes, which they donated to the Quaker Library at the Friends House in Euston. Nothing more is known of the fate of Trains No. 3 and No. 10, but No. 16 was sent east at the end of the war and used to repatriate Russian POWs from Germany. Many of its wartime staff continued to serve on board. The train was finally decommissioned in 1921 and returned to civilian commuter service in Britain.

All army chaplains were instructed to hold a service of thanksgiving on 17 November 1918. **Ernest Crosse** was particularly relieved when the Armistice was declared. He never told his family, but he believed that had the Allies lost the war, he might have lost his faith in God altogether. By the end of the war he was in Italy, and he spent all night cycling to a printer's to have 5,000 copies of a hymn sheet produced, which he distributed during a whole day of thanksgiving services held in camp after camp.[10] On his return to England he became Canon of Chichester Cathedral and headmaster at Ardingly School. He later went back to parish work, first in Henley-on-Thames and then in Glynde in East Sussex. Crosse wrote three books on chaplaincy and war, and his artefacts from the Somme – including the map on which he had marked the graves of the soldiers he had buried – were shown in the Imperial War Museum's 2009 exhibition, 'War and Memory'.

One by one, the other padres came home and continued their ministries.[11] **Wilfred Abbott** went to the Transvaal, before returning to Britain to serve at St Paul's, Haggerston in the East End of London. He retired to Brighton in 1938. **John Murray** returned to his parish in Southwark and died in 1943. **Montagu Bere** went to Shanklin in Portsmouth, where he remained until his retirement in 1935. **Cyril Horsley-Smith** stayed in France until 1920, working with a huge parish of bored soldiers waiting to be demobbed. In 1929 he took his daughter to France to show her where he had served, including a cemetery where he had buried every single man lying there. It was some consolation to him that the graves were consecrated as he had left them and were well looked after. Horsley-Smith had four parishes between 1930 and 1947, when he finally retired. He died in 1954.

None of the soldiers who had seen Father **John Lane Fox** burying men at Loos ever forgot the sight, and many of those who had known him described the chaplain as the most extraordinary man they had ever met. Father John was almost killed in 1916 when a grenade accidentally exploded and severely injured his face and right hand. At the time there was the perception that the Sacrament could not be administered by a priest with a severe physical imperfection, and Father John was devastated and feared the loss of his priestly identity. He was sent home to London to recuperate, and when his family visited him in hospital they found him on the brink of total despair, flinching at every loud noise and unable to walk without help.[12] By the time news of the Somme offensives reached the hospital he had slowly begun to recover, but his spirits only fully returned when he received confirmation from the Church authorities that Canon Law did not prevent him from officiating at Mass. By October 1916 he was back in France, where he celebrated Mass for three battalions of the Irish Guards, his broken hand holding up the Sacrament.

He remained in France for a further year, when his Order recalled him to open their new monastery at Fort Augustus in Scotland. He reluctantly obeyed and stayed in Scotland until early 1918, when he convinced the abbot to let him return to the war. He then served in Italy with the 23rd Division and took part in the battle of Vittorio Veneto. Conditions at the front were dreadful and Father John became severely ill and was sent back to the infirmary at Fort Augustus. After the war he rarely spoke about his service at the front, and it was only much later that he came to understand something of how much he had meant to the men in his care. His vocation and service gave him great joy until the end of his life. Once he was asked if he had heard of the contemporary hymn 'Lord of the Dance'; he replied that he often sang it to himself in his rooms at Fort Augustus.[13] He died there in 1974, aged ninety-four, and was buried in the abbey's cemetery on the shores of the loch. His few possessions were passed on to his family, including a chalice given to him by the Irish Guards. Small enough to be tucked into a tunic belt for use in the field, it is engraved around the base with Father John's battle honours, as proudly displayed as on any regimental flag, for the man who won them all by his love: Festubert 1915 – Loos 1915 – Somme 1916 – Ypres 1917 – Lille 1918.

Without **Claire Tisdall**'s memoir, the London Ambulance Column would have disappeared from history. But she too was a casualty with invisible scars, and it took her decades to find the strength to revisit her wartime experience. In early 1919 she caught flu and then suffered a nervous breakdown. By 1923 she had recovered sufficiently to take up a place at King's College to study for a much longed-for undergraduate degree in medieval English literature; she graduated in 1927 with a 2.1. Nothing more is known about her life until the late 1960s, when she retired to the small village of Ringmer in Sussex. Incidentally, Ernest Crosse was rector in the next village along the Downs, Glynde, at the same time, but there is no evidence that they ever met. In Ringmer she began her memoir, writing with the clarity and skill of an English scholar, although she was never able to quite purge the text of the deep, unmended pain. She completed her LAC memoir in 1976 and sent a copy for storage in the archives of the Imperial War Museum. Claire Tisdall died sometime in the early 1980s, in the shadow of the Sussex Downs. One more life given to the war, finally at peace.

Acknowledgements

First and foremost, my thanks go to the staff of the Library and Archives at the Imperial War Museum. In particular, I am grateful to Jane Smith, whose inspirational searches provided me with a number of precious sources. Geoff Bridger, battlefield historian, was extremely generous in sharing with me unpublished material on the battle of Neuve Chapelle. His wife, Anna Mae Bridger, and her colleagues at the Ringmer Historical Society were similarly helpful and generous with their time, tracking down memories of Claire Tisdall in their village. Dr Roderick Bailey found a number of original sources for me, including the bearers' map on the endpapers of this book, and listened patiently over a number of years as the work evolved. Christian Dinesen read every draft and was unfailingly supportive and calm. Likewise Dr Colin Hughes, who offered guidance and expertise throughout and directed me to the Oxford Digital Archive. Neil Taylor's expertise was also greatly appreciated.

Invaluable technical assistance came from a variety of people. Dr Annabel Emslie made sure that my understanding of early twentieth-century anaesthetics was up to snuff. Dr Tom David carefully explained military scientific and medical research. Robert Mayhew advised on details of cross-Channel weather and distances, and on the keeping of ferrets. Rob Burkett and Major (Retd) Vince Ward shared their knowledge of the life of Charles Valadier. Mr Frank Tips of the Belgian Blues ensured that that my spelling and pronunciation of Belgian place names were correct.

British historians are truly lucky in the range of archives and resources available to them and in the expertise of the men and women who work there. Susan McGann, from the Archives of the Royal College of Nursing in Edinburgh, enabled me to discover the provision made for exhausted nurses during the Great War. Sebastian Wormell, the archivist at Harrods, was hugely helpful in his provision of material from wartime catalogues and on Harrods' staff contacts in France. Captain Pete Starling of the Army Medical Services Museum was an excellent and enthusiastic guide to the library and archives; the museum may be small, but it is first-rate. Mrs P. Hatfield of the Eton College Library sought out material on the Dent family for me, and Michael Palmer, archivist at the Zoological Society of London, explained what FRZS meant in 1918. I also commend Mr Andrew Bamji, founder and steward of the Gillies Archive at Sidcup, who has preserved material that would otherwise have been lost and has done the history of medicine a great service. The librarians at Lambeth Palace, who dug out one *Crockford's* after another for me, are also thanked here, as are those at the Royal College of Surgeons in Lincoln's Inn Field.

The chapter on chaplains at the front would have been quite impossible without contributions from the following people. Dr Michael Snape, of the University of Birmingham, gave me an opportunity to try out my material at the Amport House Conference in 2009. He was extremely supportive of the research I was undertaking and provided me with a number of crucial sources. Dr Edward Madigan, of Trinity College, Dublin, explained the complexities of Catholic nomenclature and pastoral relations to me, as well as providing references from his own work. The Ven. William Jacob, Archdeacon of Charing Cross, was similarly helpful with the detail of Canon Law and other clerical detail. Polly McKay referred me to Clive Castle of St Luke's Church in Bath, who kindly found the photograph of Chaplain Doudney, his memorial and his obituary in the parish magazine. He also provided copies of the parish newsletter for me. David Black of the Museum of Army Chaplaincy was a great source of useful information and support, and in particular gave me details of the changed curriculum for chaplains in 1917. Father Timothy Radcliffe, OM, gave up an afternoon to share with me his memories of his godfather, Dom John Lane Fox. He also illuminated my understanding of service and ministry, as well as providing me with photographs and other material without which the chapter on chaplains would be much the poorer. In addition, he referred me to Robin Baird-Smith, who generously gave me copies of his correspondence with Dom John as well as great insight into the direction of the work. Our Imperial College Chaplain, Andrew Wilson, read the chapter and improved it with his clear, detailed comments.

Bert Payne's granddaughter, Sarah Pickstone, directed me to his sound archive with all its wonderful, heart-stopping detail. She also found his photograph for me and shared her memories for the Epilogue. Dr Sanders Marble, Senior Historian of the Office of Medical History for the US Army, has given me countless opportunities to talk over details, themes and historiography relating to the Great War. His expertise and thoughtfulness were crucial in shaping the material in this book. Dr Jessica Reinisch of Birkbeck College translated chunks of German for me at very short notice. Thanks go also to Dr Claire Elliott for her perceptive questions and observations about the physical and spiritual traces of the Great War on the body and psyche of the nation.

Finally, it has been a great privilege to work with Jenny Stephens and the extraordinary artists of the Birmingham Repertory Theatre as they prepared the play *Wounded* using sections of research and analysis from my chapter on stretcher bearers. Their skill and commitment to the material, and their brilliant performances, were astonishing, and it was a privilege to watch them bring history to life. Thank you all.

Notes and References

Introduction

These notes are intended for those readers who wish to go beyond the main narrative of *Wounded* to connect directly with the primary sources and the context of their production. They give detailed references for each source and also provide a brief commentary on current academic analysis and historiography, with details of related secondary literature. They examine shifts in interpretation and, in places, suggest areas where further research is required.

Wounded does not have a conventional bibliography, but there are four key works of medical history that constitute an analytical framework for the book. Mark Harrison's *The Medical War: British Military Medicine in the First World War* (Oxford University Press, 2010), Jeffrey Reznick's *Healing the Nation: Soldiers and the Culture of Caregiving in Britain during the Great War* (Manchester University Press, 2004) and Christine Hallett's *Containing Trauma: Nursing Work in the First World War* (Manchester University Press, 2009) are specialist academic histories that focus on a range of specific themes and contexts, including developments in public health, social and political attitudes to the care of the fighting soldier, and the skills and status of nurses in the period. Ian Whitehead's *Doctors in the Great War* (Leo Cooper, 1999) remains the standard account of the war's impact on the medical profession. These four works come with extensive bibliographies which, taken together, provide an almost definitive list of secondary sources for the study of medicine in the Great War. For a general overview, John Keegan's *The First Word War* (Pimlico, 1999) sets the standard for efficient and clear military history.

In 1914, the Royal Army Medical Corps had 20,000 personnel of all ranks and 7,000 hospital beds. Although medics had information on casualty treatment during the Russo-Japanese War of 1904–5, it was not thought to be relevant, so the Boer War in South Africa remained the model for military medical services. Preparations were made on this basis, even though some senior medics, such as Sir Frederick Treves, feared they would be inadequate.[1] Surgeons thought that gunshot casualties would have 'in-and-out' wounds, aseptic and sterile, needing nothing more than standard civilian antiseptic responses to heal without trouble. 'Never was a teaching more false', was the conclusion reached by two surgeons writing of their experiences stationed on both the Eastern and Western Fronts.[2] In a report published after the war, the Medical Research Council noted that there had been very few doctors with the right kind of experience for the wounds of the Flanders casualty, complicated as they were by infection, gangrene, a variety of shock symptoms, cold, and the agonisingly slow evacuation procedures.[3]

It wasn't just surgeons and doctors who lacked experience. The Voluntary Aid Detachment (VAD), which would send many of the nurses and orderlies to medical facilities in France, practised entraining and detraining casualties in elaborate exercises during 1913 and 1914. But these were primarily designed to attract recruits who were drawn more to the active nature of the events than to first aid courses and bandage-rolling in cold village halls.[4] Some medical officers took unilateral action. Captain Somerville Hastings analysed papers from German and French military congresses and journals to see if they contained anything useful. He privately published his findings as *First Aid for the Trenches*, but they would not be available for his colleagues until 1916, when the book was given a wider audience through publication by John Murray.

By 1918, the RAMC comprised 13,000 officers and 154,000 other ranks, including bearers and orderlies. Over the course of the war, 2.5 million wounded were brought home to Britain in 63 hospital trains and 66 hospital ships. Overall, there were 364,000 hospital beds in Britain and France, and a similar number across the Empire, all of which would be used many times over. In Britain, the war caused 11 million casualties. Forty per cent of all those who served either ended up with a disability pension or their dependants were in receipt of a death pension.

The creation of such a huge new medical system was a remarkable achievement, and this was recognised at the time. Surgeon-General Anthony Bowlby, who had served at CCS No. 38 and operated on the

Rev. Charles Doudney, favourably reviewed surgical provision in his report of 1917, 'The Development of British Surgery at the Front'.[5] The 1919 MRC report was one of the very first official sources to note the contributions of nurses to the process. But that same year senior medic Wilmot Heringham wrote a memoir, *A Physician in France* (Edward Arnold, 1919), which lamented the lack of recognition for the staff of the CCSs and showed concern that their extraordinary work with the wounded of the Western Front would be ignored. He was right. Over the next eighty years, records would disappear, memories would fade and the achievements of many of the medical trades involved in the care for the wounded would be marginalised. Medical histories of the war would become 'increasingly fragmented . . . [with] few works of synthesis and comparison capable of providing a rounded view of what medicine meant to their contemporaries'.[6] *Wounded* seeks to put medical history back at the heart of studies of the Great War and give credit and understanding where it is long overdue.

REFERENCES

1   See Ian Whitehead, *Doctors in the Great War* (Leo Cooper, 1999), p. 170, and Mark Harrison, *The Medical War: British Military Medicine in the First World War* (Oxford University Press, 2010).

2   B. Hughes and H. S. Banks, *War Surgery from Firing Line to Base* (Bailliere, Tindall and Cox, 1918), p. 29.

3   See Cowell and Fraser, 'A Clinical Study of the Blood Pressure in Wound Conditions', MRS Special Report No. 25, 1919.

4   See *Journal of the RAMC*, vol, 32, no. 1, 14 January 1915, p. 63 on the VAD's pre-war exercises.

5   *British Medical Journal*, 2 June 1917, pp. 705-12.

6   Harrison, *The Medical War*, p. 13.

1 Wounded

Mickey Chater was wounded at Neuve Chapelle just as the military medical system on the Western Front disintegrated. Both the nature of his wounds and his only battle set a pattern for the remainder of the war. The trauma to Chater's body was unprecedentedly severe and complex, brutally demonstrating the effect of the war's new weapons. Bullets and fragments of shell had both primary and secondary wounding power within seconds of impact. In Chater's case, whatever struck his face had enough force to cross from one cheekbone to the other. As it hit hard bone, its power was transmitted around Chater's whole upper jaw, blowing it away and battering his nose into pieces.

Every bullet or shell fragment that hit a soldier on the Western Front had the same potential for destruction. In *White Heat: The New War, 1914–1918* (Sidgwick & Jackson, 1982) John Terraine describes the technological developments that underpinned the conduct of the war. He argues that artillery significantly changed the battlefield: 'Artillery was the battle-winner, artillery was what caused the greatest loss of life, the most dreadful wounds, the deepest fear.' Terraine's work is a careful analysis of how new weaponry and technology had primarily strategic and tactical but also physical consequences.

Chater's archive at the Imperial War Museum (ref. 87/56/1) is rich and well organised. He had enthusiastically joined the war in 1914 and witnessed the Christmas Truce. After his wounding his memoirs focus on his injuries, their medical treatment and the commitment of his doctors as they struggled to restore him.

REFERENCES

1   Papers of Marie Chisholm, archives of the IWM, 01/42/1.

2   A. E. Francis, *History of the 2nd/3rd East Lancashire Field Ambulance* (Francis Jackson, 1930), p. 133.

3   See Cyril Falls, *The Gordon Highlanders in the First World War* (University of Aberdeen Publications, 1974), p. 38.

4   2nd Lt C. G. Tennant, letter to his wife, 21 March 1915, archives of the IWM, 68/12/1.

5   See Geoff Bridger, *The Battle of Neuve Chapelle* (Leo Cooper, 2000), and John Keegan, *The First World War* (Pimlico, 1999).

6   John Terraine, *White Heat: The New War, 1914–1918* (Sidgwick & Jackson, 1982), p. 146.

7   The new ammunition could have particularly devastating effects on the human face: 'High velocity bullets at short range, traversing the face approximately from one malar region to another. Encountering hard bone on the way, its force is transmitted to the

upper jaw, detaching it from its superior attachment. The whole support of the nose is also destroyed.' Mickey Chater would experience a very similar wound to the one described here by Harold Gillies in *Plastic Surgery of the Face* (Frowde, 1920), p. 226.

8   2nd Lt C. G. Tennant, letter to his wife, 21 March 1915.

9   Very few of the medics and surgeons in France had any experience of severe facial wounds. They were not unprecedented, however: similar kinds of casualty had occurred during the American Civil War. One surgeon, Dr Gurdon Buck, who treated many such cases, photographed his patients for an illustrated textbook, *Contributions to Reparative Surgery* (New York, 1876). It had been available in Britain, but was considered to be so gruesome that it might put medics off war service. See A. J. Bollet, *Civil War Medicine* (Galen Press, 2002).

10 See the papers of Dorothy Seymour, archives of the IWM, 95/28/1, entry for 15 March 1915.

11 Francis, *History*, p. 133.

ART

Joseph Gray, *A Ration Party of the 4th Black Watch at the Battle of Neuve Chapelle, 1915*; Gilbert Rogers, *A British Red Cross Society and Order of St John of Jerusalem Motor Driver*. Henry Tonks's pastels of facial casualties illustrate similar injuries and surgical reconstructions to those suffered by Mickey Chater.

POETRY

There was larksong just as the first barrage rang out at Neuve Chapelle, and the sound of birdsong on the battlefield always came as a surprise to the soldiers on the Western Front. See Isaac Rosenberg, 'Returning, we hear the Larks'.

2 Bearers

The creation of a stretcher-bearer corps was the first step in rebuilding the collapsed medical system on the Western Front in 1915, just as the

bearers themselves were the first step on the journey of the wounded
to safety and medical care. Stretcher bearers gave whatever treatment
they could as soon as they found the casualty, trying to secure his
immediate survival. They then carried him safely to a fixed site of
medical provision, such as an aid post or the dugout of an RMO. This
process – where treatment was given as close to the time and place
of wounding as possible – transformed military medical provision on
the Western Front and remains the standard in the twenty-first century.

Within a year, an entire service battalion was created almost from
scratch, consisting of technically expert staff who were trained in both
Britain and France. There were more bearers than any other medical
trade in France, and they spent longer on the battlefield than anyone
else, including soldiers. Like doctors, nurses and the wounded, bearers
wrote their memoirs in the years immediately following the war. These
included Pat McGill's *The Great Push*, William St Clair's *The Road to St
Julien*, J. H. Newton's *A Stretcher Bearer's Diary*, Frank Dunham's *The
Long Carry*, and *Stretcher Bearers . . . At the Double!* by Frederick Walter
Noyes, but most are out of print and none well known.

However, if there were policy or operational documents from the
War Office or the Army Medical Services relating to the creation and
administration of the stretcher-bearer corps, they have been lost. There
are similarly no archives from the training facilities for bearers or from
the publishers of their manuals. Perhaps because of this, the stretcher
bearers are all but invisible in the Official Medical Histories of the
war, where the only mention of the word 'bearer' in the index refers
to porters in the campaign in Cameroon. It is an example of marginalisation and, in the words of Mark Harrison, of how 'the medical
world, which made such an impression on contemporaries has faded
from view'.

But such marginalisation may also have another cause. Medical
histories of the war analyse the impact of military service on the
primary medical professions and their members: surgeons, doctors
and nurses. There is almost no analysis for the auxiliary medical trades.
Yet as we have seen, auxiliaries – and stretcher bearers in particular
– were vital to the conduct of the medical war. Bearers were a separate,
defined element of the medical organisation in France. They were
specifically recruited for their post. They had codified education and
training. They had considerable technical skill, such as the control of
haemorrhages and the application of splints. They had their own

manual, which was constantly updated to take into account new types of ammunition and improvements in treatment. The use of expert bearer teams became the standard in British military medicine.

Bearers were not the only auxiliary medical trade whose history should be analysed alongside those of surgeons, doctors and nurses: there were also orderlies, anaesthetists and X-ray technicians. A pioneering work in this respect is Jeffrey Reznick's *Healing the Nation*, which among other topics discusses the work of physiotherapists at the Shepherd's Bush Military Hospital. Reznick portrays physical and occupational therapy in its own right, rather than as an adjunct to orthopaedic surgery. A full medical history of the Great War must account for all the relevant personnel involved in saving and treating the wounded, whatever their status or skills.

As *Wounded* went to press, new research was being done by Dr Jessica Mayer, who leads the medical strand of Leeds University's Legacies of War project. Her areas of analysis include the masculine identity of medical auxiliaries during the First World War, their status as non-combatant service personnel in a society engaged in total war, their dual position as uniformed members of the military and care-givers, and the relationship between RAMC auxiliaries and those serving with voluntary service units.

There is one place for researchers to go in order to (literally) hear the voices of the stretcher bearers of the Great War. The Imperial War Museum's sound archive contains a number of testimonies given directly by bearers to its historians, and that of William Easton (no. 18277) has been used here. The IWM's archives also hold the main textual sources for this chapter: the papers of Earnest Douglas (no. 6-9-1917) and William Young (no. PP/MER/90). In addition, the refer-ences below provide details of memoirs by RMOs and field ambulance personnel on which I have also drawn, to bring to life the Great War's stretcher bearers and their work.

REFERENCES

1   *Tales of a Field Ambulance: Told by Personnel* (Borough Publications, 1935), p. 68.
2   Pat McGill, *The Great Push* (Herbert Jenkins, 1916), p. 57.
3   A. E. Francis, *History of the 2nd/3rd East Lancashire Field Ambulance* (Francis Jackson, 1930), p. 87.

4   'Treatment of wounds from Fire Trench to Field Ambulance', in *Journal of the RAMC*, vol. 27, 1916, pp. 230–40.

5   Richard Chapman, IWM sound archive, no. 8578.

6   *Tales of a Field Ambulance*, p. 19.

7   Bulletin of CCS 61, item 209, archives of the IWM, Misc. 10. See also the papers of Captain Angel, archives of the IWM, 88/46/1, for details of stretcher-bearer training, especially at the Cambridge Hospital.

8   Dr Georges Dupuy, *The Stretcher Bearer* (Hodder & Stoughton, 1915). The manuals continued to be published and updated throughout the war.

9   'The Whole Duty of an RAMC Officer', *Journal of the RAMC*, vol. 32, 1916, p. 289.

10   RMO Charles McKerrow noted how bearer performance improved after every single lecture and he thoroughly approved of the new system. See the papers of Charles McKerrow, archives of the IWM, 93/20/1, entry for 30 August 1915.

11   J. H. Newton, *A Stretcher Bearer's Diary* (Stockwell, 1932), pp. 29–30.

12   *Tales of a Field Ambulance*, p. 62.

13   See McGill, *The Great Push*, p. 207.

14   William St Clair, *The Road to St Julien* (Leo Cooper, 2004), p. 36.

15   The papers of William Harris, archives of the IWM, no. 6732/78/4/1, entry for 13 November 1916.

16   Wilfred Cook, 'The Lengthened Shadow', unpublished ms, archives of the IWM, 11/7(BY).

17   Eventually the training trenches at Étaples were filled in and a large cemetery took their place, which was painted by John Lavery in 1919.

18   Captain Angel also told of being trapped in a shell hole with his patient: see papers of Captain Angel, archives of the IWM, 88/46/1.

19   *Tales of a Field Ambulance*, p. 62.

20   See Newton, *A Stretcher Bearer's Diary*, p. 22, entry for 22 July 1917. David Jones's epic poem *In Parenthesis*, set in Mametz Wood, contained the line 'But why dont [*sic*] the bastards come – / Bearers! – stret-cher bear—ers!' The simple answer is that snipers and the destruction of the terrain made it almost impossible for them to move forward.

21   Cook, 'The Lengthened Shadow'; McGill, *The Great Push*, p. 120.

Walking on the dead is an experience described by Professor Drew Gilpin Faust in her American Civil War history, *This Republic of Suffering: Death and the American Civil War* (Vintage Civil War Library, 2009), pp. 51-8.

22 St Clair, *The Road to St Julien*, p. 76. Seeing bearers pass with loaded stretchers was an image that remained with Siegfried Sassoon, who wrote of it in his poem 'Aftermath' in 1919. See Brian Gardener (ed.), *Up the Line to Death: The War Poets 1914–1918* (Methuen, 1964), p. 154.

23 R. H. Haigh and Philip Wilson Turner (eds), *The Long Carry: The Journal of Stretcher Bearer Frank Dunham* (Pergamon, 1976), p. 27.

24 McGill, *The Great Push*, p. 237.

25 *Letters of a Canadian Stretcher Bearer* (Little, Brown, 1918), p. 90.

26 See James Brady, sound archive in the IWM, 11387/2.

27 Papers of Captain Angel, entry for 29 September 1917.

28 *Tales of a Field Ambulance*, p. 49.

29 McGill, *The Great Push*, p. 145.

30 *Tales of a Field Ambulance*, p. 47. The papers of Private Herbert Empson, archive of the IWM, 02/12/1.

31 McGill, *The Great Push*, p. 143.

32 Newton, *A Stretcher Bearer's Diary*, p. 24.

33 Harold Dearden, *Medicine and Duty* (Heinemann, 1928), p. 112.

34 See *Tales of a Field Ambulance*, p. 48.

35 See *The Official History of the Medical Services of the Great War*, vol. 3, *General History*, p. 166, and St Clair, *The Road to St Julien*, p. 59.

36 *Tales of a Field Ambulance*, p. 73.

37 Ibid., p. 52.

38 Newton, *A Stretcher Bearer's Diary*, p. 74.

39 See Harold Plant, sound archive in the IWM, reel 3.

40 Joseph Yarwood, sound archive in the IWM, 12231.

41 Bernard Adams, *Nothing of Importance* (reprint; Donovan Press, 1988), p. 182.

42 St Clair, *The Road to St Julien*, p. 57. St Clair's entire division and bearer corps was shattered at Loos.

43 The poet was Geoffrey Studdert Kennedy, otherwise known as 'Woodbine Willie', who won an MC at Messines Ridge. Two hugely popular collections of his poetry were published during and just after the war: *Rough Rhymes of a Padre* and *More Rough Rhymes* (Hodder & Stoughton, 1918, 1920).

Stretcher bearers and their work made a considerable impression on the artists of the Western Front, official or otherwise, who observed important details of the skill and dedication of bearers and regarded them as worthy of the highest standards of painterly representation. Gilbert Rogers produced a whole series of drawings: *The Stretcher Bearers, A Royal Army Medical Corps Stretcher-Bearer, Fully Equipped, 'Humanity' Bearer Post, Cambrai section, August 1916: The First Field Ambulance, Stretcher Bearing in Difficulties, The Dead Stretcher Bearer* and *Ypres 1915*. In addition we have Harold Williamson's *Removing the Wounded 60 yards from the Enemy*, Charles McKay's *Portrait of a Stretcher Bearer on Water Duty*, Christopher Nevinson's *The Harvest of Battle*, P. Watkins's *An Ambulance Dressing Station on the Western Front* and Hayden McKay's *Portrait of a BRCS and Order of St John Stretcher Bearer, An RAMC Squad with Infantry: Night at Nurlu, October 1918*.

POETRY

David Jones, *In Parenthesis*; Siegfried Sassoon, 'Aftermath'; Isaac Rosenberg, 'Dead Man's Dump'; Robert Graves, 'A Child's Nightmare'.

3 Regimental Medical Officers

Two academic works provide the background for this chapter. Mark Harrison's *The Medical War* examines in detail RMOs' responsibility for the public-health aspects of medical provision in the Great War. This included the maintenance of the overall health of their battalion, such as personal and dental hygiene, sewerage and water provision, and the treatment of general ailments. Harrison's analysis links their work to broader themes of public health, military organisation and civilian expectations of medical provision for soldiers, which had evolved in the late nineteenth century. Ian Whitehead's *Doctors in the Great War* looks at medical provision from the point of view of the medical profession itself. Whitehead describes the impact on both the profession and their patients of the removal of so many medics from civilian life. He also examines the differences between the career RAMC doctors and their civilian volunteer colleagues, as well as their recruitment and training. Both historians come to a similar conclusion: that, despite a lack of preparation and structure, medical provision during the Great War was a success.

In this chapter the work of RMOs is described primarily in terms of their care of wounded men. Emphasis is placed on the high level of independence given to each medical officer, so that he could make his own preparations and decisions on how best to treat the wounded. This meant not only choosing the location of his aid post, but also training his stretcher-bearer teams to the highest standard possible to support his efforts. RMOs were able to set up formal and informal networks, such as the Rouen Medical Society, which was created to share knowledge and provide support. In addition there were numerous local medical societies that regularly met close to the front. The *Journal of the Royal Army Medical Corps* was fundamental to the exchange of information and experience; much of its content from 1914 to 1918 remains to be explored and analysed by historians, as do the activities and output of the Western Front's medical societies.

Although the RAMC's service records for the war no longer exist, many medical officers wrote memoirs that provide insight into both personal experience and medical policy. This chapter draws on the memoirs and papers of four RMOs, who were either GPs or surgeons in civilian life: John Linnell (unpublished manuscript, private collection), Geoffrey Hardwick (IWM, no. 98/12/4) and Charles McKerrow (IWM, no. 93/20/1); my account of William Kelsey Fry draws on Harold Gillies's *Principles and Art of Plastic Surgery* (Frowde, 1920), Siegfried Sassoon's *Memoirs of an Infantry Officer* (Faber & Faber, 1937), Joseph Hone's *The Life of Henry Tonks* (Heinemann, 1939) and obituaries of Kelsey Fry in the *Lancet*, *The Times* and the *Supplement to the London Gazette*.

REFERENCES

1   *Supplement to the London Gazette*, 24 July 1915, p. 7281.
2   See www.1914–1918.net/Diaries/wardiary-2welsh.htm, accessed 6 November 2008.
3   *Supplement to the London Gazette*, 16 November 1915, p. 11426.
4   For a full discussion of this aspect of medical care in the Great War, see Mark Harrison, 'War, Health and Citizenship: Preventative Medicine on the Western Front', in *The Medical War* (Oxford

University Press, 2010), pp. 123–70. RMOs were increasingly well trained and prepared for all aspects of service at the Officers' School of Instruction run by the RAMC. Very few records of this institution remain; some of the most useful are the painted representations of John Hodgson Lobley. His work shows that RMOs were trained to build and operate incinerators and that the training camp in Blackpool was tented, so they were prepared for life under canvas in France. Lobley's work is in the IWM art holdings, nos 3731, 3681, 3968.

5   See the papers of Major R. C. Ozanne, archives of the IWM, no. 91/23/1, entry for 21 September 1915. See also William G. MacPherson, in *The Official History of the Medical Services of the Great War*, vol. 1, *General History*, p. 150, cited in R. L. Atenstaedt, 'The Organisation of the RAMC during the Great War', in *Journal of the RAMC*, vol. 152, 2006, pp. 81–5.

6   See R. H. Haigh and Philip Wilson Turner (eds), *The Long Carry: The Journal of Stretcher Bearer Frank Dunham* (Pergamon, 1976), p. 140.

7   See Bernard Adams, *Nothing of Importance* (reprint; Donovan Press, 1988), p. 270. Bernard Adams served as an officer with the 12th and 1st Battalions of the Royal Welch Fusiliers during the First World War. The book was written as a description of his life as an infantryman whilst convalescing from wounds received during the battle of the Somme in 1916. He rejoined the 1st Battalion in February 1917 and was killed within three weeks.

8   Ibid., p. 272.

9   *Supplement to the London Gazette*, 11 March 1916, p. 2718.

10 See Siegfried Sassoon, *Memoirs of an Infantry Officer* (Faber & Faber, 1937), p. 330.

11 Ibid., pp. 376–7.

12 J. S. G. Blair, *A Centenary History of the Royal Army Medical Corps* (Lynx Publications, 2001), p. 148.

13 On the 'Year of Battles', see John Keegan, *The First World War* (Pimlico, 1999), pp. 277–331.

14 See the papers of Captain F. G. Chandler, archives of the IWM, 19 July 1916.

15 From 1917 onwards, some CCSs retained the 'so-called shell shock cases . . . in [wards] especially organised for their treatment in as advanced a position as possible'. *The Official History of the Medical Services of the Great War*, vol. 3, *General History*, p. 119.

16   Ferret-keeping was enormously popular at the time. See the Rev.
      J. W. H. Heslop, 'How to make a ferret court', in *The Boy's Own
      Paper*, 1916, p. 761.
17   'The Whole Duty of an RAMC Officer', *Journal of the RAMC*, vol.
      32, 1916, p. 289.
18   See Isaac Rosenberg, 'Dead Man's Dump', in Andrew Motion
      (ed.), *First World War Poems* (Faber and Faber, 2003).
19   See Basil Peacock, *The Royal Northumberland Fusiliers* (Leo Cooper,
      1970), and John Keegan, *The First World War* (Pimlico, 1999), pp.
      318–19.
20   C. K. McKerrow, 'Pyrexias of Doubtful Origin in an Infantry
      Battalion on Active Service', *Journal of the RAMC*, vol. 30, 1918,
      pp. 175–85.

ART

Haydn Reynolds McKay: *The Main Dressing Station of a Field Ambulance,
Templeux la Fosse, 18th September, 1918*; *Epehy: In a Sunken Roadway near
the Regimental Aid Post of the 7th Battalion Royal Sussex Regiment*; *A
British Red Cross Society and Order of St John of Jerusalem Officer in France*;
An Advanced Dressing Station for the 36th Field Ambulance at Lieramont;
and *An Advanced Dressing Station, France: Cars supplied by the British Red
Cross*.

4 Surgeons

Apart from shell shock, surgery is the most thoroughly researched
subject in the medical history of the Great War. In the Official
Histories, produced from 1922 onwards, surgery has two volumes to
itself. Leading surgeons such as Harold Gillies wrote sections on their
individual disciplines – in Gillies's case, facial repair – summarising
their work and achievements during the war. These sections aimed
to educate civilian specialists, although no hospital department was
likely to encounter injuries of similar severity or scale. The volumes
also dealt with areas related to surgery, such as blood transfusions,
anaesthesia (not yet anaesthesiology) and infections, and included long
sections on the new weaponry and its wounding effects. There was
a well-intentioned section that examined wounding by modern

artillery ('The Results of Projectile Action') but for today's reader the effect is undermined by the author's use of examples from Big Game hunting to demonstrate wounding power.

Modern historians have also paid close attention to surgery in the Great War and have put it into the broader context of industrial society. Works such as Roger Cooter's *Surgery and Society in Peace and War* (Palgrave Macmillan, 1993) compare the demands made on orthopaedic surgeons by the Great War with those of the industrial injuries generated by the building of the Manchester Ship Canal. In both cases surgeons used their much-increased caseloads to generate recognition for their specialisation and to consolidate their status. In a similar vein, Joel Howell, 'Soldier's Heart: The Redefinition of Heart Disease and Speciality Formation in Early Twentieth-Century Great Britain', in Roger Cooter, Mark Harrison and Steve Sturdy (eds), *War, Medicine and Modernity* (Sutton, 1998), focuses on heart disease in Great War soldiers and its influence on the development of cardiology. The focus of these works is broad but primarily about surgeons and dedicated units based well to the rear or in Britain. Thus the war is seen as a contributing factor in the overall development of civilian medical practice, creating the modern disciplines we recognise today.

This chapter takes a different perspective on the surgical achievements during the Great War. Even if he was a specialist in civilian life, a surgeon at the Western Front was expected to perform all types of operations, usually on an emergency basis. During battle the surgeons at the CCSs worked in theatre all day and all night, performing everything from abdominal procedures, bone-setting and amputations to arterial repair, debridement and even some basic brain surgery. This was not the frenzied hacking practised in the surgical tents in the American Civil War; it was modern surgery, with antiseptic procedures, anaesthetics and post-operative care. This chapter therefore describes an unconventional yet crucial medical breakthrough: the discovery that surgery could be done in a forward medical unit close to the actual place of wounding, and that by doing so survival rates would be radically improved. *Wounded* shifts the attention back onto developments in military, rather than civilian medicine. What was created at the Western Front was nothing less than a new model for military surgery and military medical care.

The chapter uses three primary sources. Henry Souttar's *A Surgeon in Belgium* (Edward Arnold, 1915) is one of the few memoirs to describe in detail the setting up of a forward surgical facility in the early months of the war. By the time Norman Pritchard wrote his diaries (IWM, no. 03/17/1) the CCS was established as the centrepiece of medical provision in France. John Hayward (www.firstworldwar.com/ diaries/casualtyclear ingstation.htm, accessed 27 October 2010) was a CCS surgeon in the last summer of the war, when the military medical facilities were at a high point in terms of numbers, skill and range of provision.

REFERENCES

1   Hartnell Beavis and Henry Souttar, 'A Field Hospital in Belgium', *British Medical Journal*, 9 January 1915, p. 66.

2   Sir Henry Sessions Souttar features in the *Oxford Dictionary of National Biography* (Oxford University Press, 2004), entry no 36303, written by Tom Treasure.

3   Sarah MacNaughtan, *My War Experiences in Two Continents*, ch. 11. 'We Go to Furnes' (BiblioBazaar reprint, 2009).

4   Beavis and Souttar, 'A Field Hospital in Belgium', pp. 64–6.

5   The nurse who couldn't stand the pressure at No. 1 Belgian Field was May Sinclair. Her despair permeates her memoir of the place, *A Journal of Impressions in Belgium* (Hutchinson, 1915). She described the hospital as 'a world apart, a world of insufferable space and agonizing time, ruled over by some inhuman mathematics and given over to pre-transcendent pain' (p. 46).

6   See Baroness de T'Serclaes, *Flanders and Other Fields* (Harrap, 1964), p. 59.

7   For details of these techniques developed by nurses in all the CCSs, see Christine E. Hallett, *Containing Trauma: Nursing Work in the First World War* (Manchester University Press, 2009).

8   *A War Nurse's Diary* (Macmillan, 1918), p. 63.

9   Elizabeth, Queen of the Belgians was profoundly interested in medicine – her German father preferring the profession of ophthalmologist to his ducal birthright. The queen drove provision for refugee Belgian servicemen almost single-handedly, raising funds, supervising building works and even nursing when necessary. See A. Nicholas, *Elizabeth Queen of the Belgians: Her Life and Times* (New Horizon, 1982), and Marie José, *Albert et Élisabeth de Belgique: Mes Parents* (Plon, 1971).

10   Both French and British medical radiology units had been
      dependent on German X-ray bulbs before the war, so it took
      some time for suppliers and manufacturers to catch up. See
      Medicine and Surgery in the Great War, catalogue of the exhibition
      held at the Wellcome Institute, 1968, and *A War Nurse's Diary*, pp.
      112, 113. For details of Curie's work at the front, see Eve Curie,
      Madame Curie: A Biography (Da Capo Press, 2001), pp. 291–302.

11   Although Curie didn't mind the tent, she was glad to be out of
      it. After Furnes, she went to a hospital in Poperinghe, from where
      she wrote to her daughter Irène that she had 'a nice room and
      they gave me a fire in a stove at the side. I'm better off than at
      Furnes.' Marie Curie to Irène Curie, from *Correspondance* (Les
      Editeurs français réunis, 1974), p. 158.

12   The story of Curie and her travelling radiographers is also covered
      in a recent work of fiction, Jeb Rubenfeld's *The Death Instinct*
      (Headline Review, 2011).

13   On the development of the CCS between 1915 and 1917, see Mark
      Harrison, *The Medical War: British Military Medicine in the First
      World War* (Oxford University Press, 2010), pp. 34–8.

14   See 'Treatment of Wounds in RAPs and FAs of the Second Army',
      regulations from the ADMS, issued 6 June 1917: 'Amputations
      should only be performed for completely shattered limbs', section
      5, p. 1 (author's collection).

15   William G. MacPherson, *Official History of the Medical Services of
      the Great War*, vol. 3, *General History*, p. 177. Amputation rates in
      civilian practice had fallen significantly as conservative surgery
      became more effective. The volume and severity of femoral frac-
      tures caused by bullet and shell fragments was a challenge to this
      new methodology. Most surgeons amputated when confronted
      with a femoral fracture in the hospitals in France, which was felt
      to be the only solution to avoid death from gas gangrene or blood
      loss. In 1917 more effective splinting of compound fractures was
      introduced and amputation rates fell dramatically in the last year
      of the war. Stretcher bearers were trained to use the new Thomas
      Splint, which was simple and effective. In particular, the splint
      could be applied over uniform rags, so was quick and easy to use
      even under fire. Ironically, by 1918 many of the splints being used
      by bearer teams and MOs on the Western Front had been manu-
      factured in occupational-health rehabilitation centres by disabled

or amputee soldiers retraining for civilian life. See P. M. Robinson and M. J. O'Meara, 'The Thomas Splint: Its Origins and Use in Trauma', *Journal of Bone and Joint Surgery*, April 2009, vol. 91-B, pp. 540–54, and John Kirkup, *A History of Limb Amputation* (Springer, 2007), p. 92. For details of the occupational therapy that manufactured splints and other medical items, see Jeffrey S. Reznick, *Healing the Nation: Soldiers and the Culture of Caregiving in Britain During the Great War* (Manchester University Press, 2004), pp. 116–37.

16 See the papers of Captain Fred Chandler, archives of the IWM, 07/21/1, correspondence of 7 November 1917.

17 See Georges Duhamel, *The New Book of Martyrs* (William Heinemann, 1918) p. 58. For details of both the technical difficulties of early anaesthetics and an unusual female anaesthetist, see Hanine Fourie, 'The Untold Story of a Great War Anaesthetist: Lady Helen D'Abernon', unpublished research essay, May 2009, available in the Imperial College Library. See also Helen Venetia Vincent D'Abernon, 'War Case-book, 1915–1918', archives of the IWM, 92/22/1.

18 For the immediate results of the war experience on the surgical profession, see George H. Makins, 'Introductory', *British Journal of Surgery* (special issue), 1918, vol. VI, no. 21, pp. 1–11.

ART

John Hodgson Lobley, *The Operating Theatre, First Casualty Clearing Station*, Christopher Nevinson, *The Doctor* and *Night Arrival*; John Singer Sargent, *Gassed*; Henry Tonks, *An Advanced Dressing Station in France*, *An Underground Casualty Clearing Station, Arras* and *A Saline Infusion*.

POETRY

Wilfred Owen, 'Conscious'; Vera Brittain, 'The German Ward'.

5 Wounded

Bert Payne's testimony was given directly to the IWM's sound archive (no. 9894) and has been supplemented by information from his family.

The main source for the material on the first day of the battle of the Somme is Martin Middlebrook's *The First Day of the Somme* (Penguin, 2006). Detail on the nature and flavour of octanes and caffeine was supplied by students of the Imperial College Chemistry Department.

ART

Henry Tonks's collection of pastel drawings of facial casualties; John Hodgson Lobley's *Wounded Passing through Snow Hill Railway Station, Birmingham*.

6 Nurses

The history of nurses and nursing in the Great War, like that of surgeons and surgery, is a field that has generated interest and research continually since the end of the war. Historical studies of nursing in the twentieth century have focused on the influence of war on the development and status of the profession. These works also emphasise the broader social context of wartime nursing: suffragism, the campaigns for women's rights and the changing expectations of the public role of women in the period. Some studies have looked at femininity in the context of industrialised warfare. In addition to these academic studies, nurses wrote some of the finest memoirs of the Great War. Vera Brittain's *Testament of Youth* is the most famous, but less well-known memoirs by Olive Dent and K. E. Luard also provide unique insight into life and service at the front and have been used in *Wounded*.

In the twenty-first century, historians have begun to take a different path by looking closely at the technical aspects of wartime nursing. Christine Hallett's *Containing Trauma* is an entirely new representation of the work of nurses at the front and draws out subtle, essential detail about the precise nature of their achievements and skills. Hallett describes the complexity of nursing care: how technical medical knowledge was fused with attention to the whole patient who was recovering or beyond recovery. Moreover, she judges these skills in their own right, not as adjuncts to surgery, and reveals how nursing skills and experience facilitated the development of the CCS as a clinically capable forward medical facility. Hallett's emphasis on the expertise of nurses at the CCSs in France matches the focus of *Wounded*.

Nurses' memoirs are some of the most valuable testimonies of all the medical staff on the Western Front. Not only do they describe their work with the wounded, but they provide some of the most detailed descriptions of the CCSs themselves and what it was like to live and work immersed in the war. CCSs had no facilities to produce notes and reports or to store archive material, so there is very little information about individual units in the official records. Nurses' memoirs fill in many of the gaps. We learn, for example, that most CCSs had a rich and varied social life that included concerts and fancy-dress competitions. The nurses' frankness about how the war engulfed and threatened to overwhelm them, however, reveals the limits of even the most advanced military medical system.

In addition, these memoirs often hint at the psychological trauma suffered by medical personnel serving in the Great War. Nurses in particular needed periods of rest away from their post, which was provided by Queen Mary's Army Auxiliary Corps Home for Convalescents in France and the Edith Cavell Homes in Britain. Some nurses recovering there had been so badly affected by their experiences that they never returned to the front. The toll that the war took on all ranks of medical personnel at the Western Front could be severe, but to date there is no body of research comparable to that on shell shock which investigates its consequences. Much more work is needed, and nurses' memoirs would be an excellent place to start.

There are three primary sources for this section, all from the archives of the Imperial War Museum. Sister Jentie Patterson (ref. 90/10/1) describes how a CCS that dispensed hot drinks and fresh dressings to casualties was converted into a fully fledged forward hospital, while Winifred Kenyon (ref. 84/24/1) provides great insight into daily life at one of the new expert CCSs. Nurse Elizabeth Boon's contribution is her letter to the family of Private Simpson (ref. Misc. 262/5562), which draws together many of the themes of this chapter about the unique contribution made by nurses to the medical care at the Western Front.

REFERENCES

1   See H. S. Souttar, *A Surgeon in Belgium* (Edward Arnold, 1915) p. 18.

2   See the papers of No. 61 Casualty Clearing Station, archives of the IWM, Misc 10, item 209, 17/7/18.

3   Olive Dent, *A VAD Nurse in France* (Grant Richards, 1917), p. 263.

4   Ibid., p. 61.

5   K. E. Luard, *Unknown Warrior* (Chatto & Windus, 1930) p. 8.

6   See Bernard Adams, *Nothing of Importance* (reprint; Donovan Press, 1988).

7   Dent, *A VAD Nurse in France,* p. 47.

8   Ibid., p. 279.

9   Lady Helen D'Abernon, *Red Cross and Berlin Embassy* (John Murray, 1946), p. 32.

10 Dent, *A VAD Nurse in France,* p. 140.

11 Ibid., p. 329.

12 There were also convalescent homes in Britain for nurses who broke under the strain. The first Edith Cavell Home of Rest for Nurses was opened in November 1917, with Elizabeth, Queen of the Belgians as patron. Its aim was 'the establishment of Homes of temporary rest for practising trained women, nurses and practitioners, who are or who have been employed in civil or military hospitals or in connection with the war or in any other capacity whatever and have become temporarily in need of mental of physical rest'. See Christine E. Hallett, *Containing Trauma: Nursing Work in the First World War* (Manchester University Press, 2009), p. 215; see also papers relating to The Nation's Fund for Nurses in the archives of the Wellcome Trust, SA/NFN/C/1.2.

13 Dent, *A VAD Nurse in France,* p. 333.

14 See Susan Richmond, 'Little Short of a Miracle', *History Today,* July 2006, pp. 12–21.

15 Alexandrina Marsden, *Resistance Nurse* (Odhams Press, 1961), p. 48.

16 See D'Abernon, *Red Cross and Berlin Embassy,* p. 27.

17 Dent, *A VAD Nurse in France,* p. 270.

18 Ibid., p. 313.

19 *A War Nurse's Diary* (Macmillan, 1918), p. 109.

20 Dent, *A VAD Nurse in France,* p. 150.

21 See the papers of F. Davison, archives of the IWM, no. 03/15/1.

22 Luard, *Unknown Warrior,* p. 68.

23 Dent, *A VAD Nurse in France,* p. 201.

24 Luard, *Unknown Warrior,* p. 163.

25 This wasn't just kindness on the nurses' part. The system was felt to be so effective that keeping a ward notebook became

official RAMC policy: 'Special care should be taken to safeguard the belongings of dying patients. Messages and wishes should be carefully recorded and a special book kept for this purpose.' See 'The Casualty Clearing Station as a Working Unit in the Field', *Journal of the RAMC*, vol. 32, 1916, p. 45.

26 Dent, *A VAD Nurse in France*, p. 284.

ART

John Lavery, *Portrait of Nurse Billam and Sister Currier* and *The Queen Mary Army Auxiliary Corps Convalescent Home, Le Touquet*; William Hatherell, *Nurse, Wounded Soldier and Child*; John Lavery, *German Wounded at Etaples*; John Hodgson Lobley, *The Camp of the 42nd Casualty Clearing Station, Douai*; William Hatherall, *The Last Message*; Martin Edwin, *The Second Casualty Clearing Station, Douai*.

POETRY

Anonymous, 'To Little Sister, No. 16'; Siegfried Sassoon, 'Died of Wounds' and 'The Deathbed'; Wilfred Gibson, 'Mark Anderson'; Wilfred Owen, 'The Dead-Beat'.

7 Orderlies

Orderlies provide further evidence for the high levels of skill and training given to the auxiliary medical trades at the Western Front. Like the stretcher bearers, their history has also faded from the record.

Two testimonies have been selected from the archives of the IWM: those of Alfred Arnold (ref. no. 9691) and Harold Foakes (ref. no. 99/54/1).

REFERENCES

1   See the papers of Private Herbert Empson of 2nd/5th Field Ambulance, 180 Infantry Brigade, in the archives of the IWM, 02/12/1.

2   See John Keegan, *The First World War* (Pimlico, 1999), pp. 350–3, for an account of the battle of Arras and its aftermath.

ART

John Hodgson Lobley, *Reception for the Wounded at the First Casualty Clearing Station, Le Chateau, during the British Advance in October 1918.*

8 Wounded

John Glubb was a prolific writer and his memoirs, produced after his retirement from the Arab Legion, were extremely popular with the public. While he appeared to have suffered little psychological trauma from his experiences in France, he spares no detail in his account of his long and often difficult recovery. *Into Battle* (Cassell, 1977) covers the period of his injury and treatment; additional details were supplied by Trevor Royle's biography, *Glubb Pasha.*

REFERENCES

1   Trevor Royle, *Glubb Pasha* (Little, Brown, 1992), p. 59.
2   Ibid., p. 60.
3   Head injuries were upsetting for everyone in the wards. They were almost always fatal and patients were noisy, incoherent, vomited frequently and had to be subdued with knockout doses of morphine. See John Laffin, *Surgeons in the Field* (Dent, 1970), p. 225.
4   See Royle, *Glubb Pasha*, p. 61.
5   Ibid., p. 62.

POETRY

Wilfred Gibson, 'In the Ambulance'.

9 Chaplains

Throughout the twentieth century the history of military chaplaincy was dominated by the issue of denomination. Historians explored the distinctions between Catholic, Anglican and Nonconformist clergy in their attitudes towards the war and the military, and have focused on the differences in their recruitment of battalion padres. In addition, Robert Graves's *Goodbye to All That* (Jonathan Cape, 1929) has had a lasting influence on our understanding of chaplaincy during the Great War. In the earliest editions of the book, chaplains across the board come in for criticism, but in later revisions Graves depicts all Anglican chaplains as cowardly fools and all Roman Catholic padres as absurdly brave and inspiring.

In recent years, however, historians have sought to broaden the focus of their research beyond issues of denomination and they have questioned the accuracy of Graves's characterisations. Drawing on clerical records and both chaplains' and soldiers' memoirs, Edward Madigan's study *Faith under Fire: Anglican Clergy and the Great War* (Palgrave Macmillan, 2011) shows that bravery and cowardice were ecumenical. Clergymen of all types could be found both on the battlefield and hiding in a tent to the rear; courage was a question of character, not denomination. Moreover, the work of Michael Snape has introduced a new analytical framework to the history of military chaplaincy. In *God and the British Soldier* (Routledge, 2005) and *Clergy under Fire* (Boydell Press, 2007), Snape has looked at the state of religion in modern Britain and how different forms of religiosity affected the morale of soldiers. He has also studied in detail the work of the Royal Army Chaplains Department and its educational facilities. Both Madigan and Snape have provided a new and invigorating basis for future work in the field.

This new work emphasises the responsibility that chaplains took for caring for the dead, particularly in ensuring that burials were proper and prompt. There is less focus on the relationships that they had with the world of the wounded. Linda Parker's *The Whole Armour of God* (Helion & Company, 2013) contains a chapter on chaplains and doctors but concentrates on the religious context of their work and provides very little medical detail. *Wounded*, by contrast, focuses on chaplains who worked in medical facilities and engaged closely with both patients and medics in a personal redefinition of their ministry. Catholic monk, Anglican vicar or Nonconformist minister, they all made the same choice: it was at aid posts, CCSs and base hospitals that their presence was most needed.

In common with all the section titles in *Wounded*, this chapter heading is deliberately simple. It gives only the names of the men whose memoirs have been studied, not their denomination or clerical

rank. Here and elsewhere in the book, commitment to the care of
the wounded is the primary concern, beyond details of rank, education, professional status or recruitment type. Each chaplain, regardless
of his background, was determined to find a place at the Western
Front where he could best serve the soldiers. Each found his way to
a medical facility, whether it was a front-line aid post, a casualty
clearing station or a base hospital to the rear.

Chaplain memoirs are a particularly rich historical source. In addition to their being educated men and used to writing, there were few
others who observed the system of medical care in all its forms and
details. Chaplains worked everywhere. They could be found in hospital
mail rooms, operating theatres or lonely outposts in no-man's-land.
They stayed for long periods in their postings and watched the medical
services around them evolving, noting the changes in their diaries.
They tell us about laboratories, post-operative wards and medical
provision for POWs. They observe how self-sufficient and multi-disci-
plinary their units became, and how expert their staff. It is a chaplain
who tells us of the new mental wards in CCSs, providing evidence
for a network of provision for shell shock and other psychological
conditions at the front. While the history of shell shock, which domi-
nates so much of the medical history of the war, focuses primarily
on treatment in Britain, such facilities in a forward position remain
under-researched. Perhaps typically, the chaplain's description of the
mental wards is coloured by his concern that he is failing to give
comfort to the patients he finds there. Although many padres felt that
they weren't doing enough, the moral authority that accrued to them
among the medical staff in France indicates otherwise.

This chapter draws primarily on personal memoirs. Wilfred Abbott's
story is told in John Linnell's unpublished memoir of the battle of
Neuve Chapelle (private collection). Ernest Crosse's extensive personal
archive is in the Imperial War Museum, where it is much used by
curators (ref. 80/22/1). Charles Doudney's life is accounted for in a
biography by his descendants, *The Best of Good Fellows* (Jonathan Home
Publications, 1995). John Murray's archive is at the IWM (ref. 77/106/1)
and additional material on him can be found in the Museum of Army
Chaplaincy at Amport House. Cyril Horsley-Smith's and Montagu
Bere's papers are also in the IWM (96/38/1 and 66/96/1 respectively).
John Lane Fox left no personal papers, but his service is recorded in
Pat MacGill's *The Great Push* (Herbert Jenkins, 1916) and in the

memories of his colleagues and relatives. I have also drawn on Owen Spencer Watkins's *With French in France and Flanders* (Kelly, 1915). This was one of the first books published by a serving chaplain and is mostly about the RAMC and the stretcher-bearer corps, both of which Spencer Watkins admired greatly. The Crockford's Clerical Directory (Church House Publishing, annually and online) provided details of the pre- and post-war lives of the chaplains in this chapter.

REFERENCES

1   See *Journal of the RAMC*, vol. 32, 1916 p. 289.

2   Owen Spencer Watkins, *With French in France and Flanders* (Kelly, 1915), p. 79. See also Michael Snape, *Clergy under Fire* (Boydell Press, 2008), pp. 190, 204 and 247. Snape also provides details of the organisation and administration of the Army Chaplains Department.

3   See Spencer Watkins, *With French in France and Flanders*, p. 79.

4   'Pending the arrival of a Medical Officer, the Reverend E. Manning will take command of the stretcher bearers, having volunteered to do so': papers of the Rev. Manning, archives of the IWM, 78/7/1/, Army Book 152, Field Despatch from Hollingsworth to DDHQ, 27 September 1917.

5   See the papers of the Rev. Mellish, archives of the IWM, PP/MCR/269. Padre Mellish won a VC at St Éloi in March 1916. See also Max Arthur's history and directory, *Symbol of Courage: A Complete History of the Victoria Cross* (Sidgwick & Jackson, 2004), p. 239.

6   Spencer Watkins, *With French in France and Flanders*, pp. 47–8, and the papers of the Very Rev. E. Milner-White, archives of the IWM, 96/38/1.

7   Ibid., p. 6, entry for 4 June 1916.

8   Ibid., p. 14.

9   Letter from Mrs Doudney to St Luke's parish magazine, Bath, May 1915. He was given donations by his parishioners for equipment that he might need in France, including a set of private Communion vessels.

10 St Luke's parish magazine, September 1908, p. 2.

11 It is perhaps not surprising that Doudney took this view of his service in France. The living at St Luke's was in the gift of the Simeon Trust, based on the teachings of the Rev. Charles Simeon, a nineteenth-century evangelical. Although Simeon believed that

conversion was at the heart of ministry, he espoused a gentler form than many of his peers, and Simeon Trust clergymen emphasised the Christian duty for social action and responsibility for one's fellow man. See the website of St Luke's Church, Wellsway, Bath, www.stlukesbath.com, accessed 20 April 2011.

12   See the papers of the Rev. L. L. Jeeves, archives of the IWM, 80/22/1. Jeeves was also mistaken for the doctor at his CCS.

13   See the papers of Canon Rogers, archives of the IWM, 77/107/1, entry for 10 March 1916. See also papers of the Rev. Dr T. H. Davies, archives of the IWM, 03/30/1, entry for 3 December 1916.

14   The papers of the Very Rev. Milner White, archives of the IWM, 96/38/1.

15   St Luke's parish newsletter, letter from Mrs Doudney, October 1915. She wrote that the vicar was having 'A nerve-shaking time – frequently up to the firing line – hiding in dug-outs to take funerals'.

16   'The Death of Charles Doudney', obituary in St Luke's parish magazine, with details from a letter by the officer commanding the 18th Field Ambulance.

17   For the 'relentless self-criticism' of some padres, see Edward Madigan's *Faith under Fire: Anglican Army Chaplains and the Great War* (Palgrave Macmillan, 2009). Madigan cites examples of chaplains who were 'painfully aware' of the limitations of their ministry and their own shortcomings as messengers for Christ, whether they worked in a medical setting or elsewhere at the front. Madigan thinks that one particularly interesting feature of the personal narratives produced by Anglican chaplains during the war was their honesty about the difficulties inherent in their ministry; author's email exchange with Dr Madigan, 22 August 2011.

18   For details of the work on these new mental wards offering 'Forward Psychiatry', see Edgar Jones, Adam Thomas and Stephen Ironside, 'Shell Shock: an outcome study of a First World War PIE unit', *Psychological Medicine*, 2007, vol. 37, pp. 215–23.

19   See 'Question XXVIII: Of Joy', in Thomas Aquinas, *Aquinas Ethicus: or, the Moral Teaching of St Thomas*, vol. 1 (Summa Theologica – Prima Secundae, Secunda Secundae Pt. 1), 1274. I am grateful to Father Timothy Radcliffe for this reference.

20   Papers of Canon F. H. Drinkwater, archives of the IWM, 99/54/1, entry for 29 August 1915: 'Those brown blankets – they will always remind me of wounds and death.'

21 The papers of Rev. Smithwick, diary entry for 25 September 1916, archives of the IWM, 01/59/1.

22 Papers of Canon F. H. Drinkwater, diary entry for 1 July 1916.

23 See *The Official Medical History of the Great War* (HMSO, 1924), vol. 3, p. 163.

24 The papers of the Reverend Wilkinson, archives of the IWM, 67/22/1.

25 Another chaplain showed an early insight into the diagnosis of shell shock that was becoming increasingly familiar: 'I am certain the shell shock was caused not just by the explosion of a shell near by but by the sights and smell and horror of the battlefield in general.' See the papers of Rev. D. Railton, archives of the IWM, 80/22/1, entry for 24 September 1916.

26 From David Blake, 'Chaplaincy Training during the First World War', *Journal of the RACD*, 2007, vol. 46, pp. 41–2.

27 For details of the 'pointless' battle of Loos, see John Keegan, *The First World War* (Pimlico, 1999), pp. 217–19.

28 Father John Lane Fox to Robin Baird-Smith, private correspondence, 12 April 1969. Father John was eighty-nine years old at the time of writing. In *The Great Push* (New York: George Doran, 1916) Pat McGill describes his grave-digging: 'Often at night the sentry on watch can see a dark form between the lines working with a shovel and spade, burying the dead. The bullets whist by, hissing of death and terror; now and then a bomb whirls in the air and bursts loudly . . . but indifferent to the clamour and tumult, the solitary digger bends over his work burying the dead.'

ART

John Hodgson Lobley, *The RAMC in Training, Blackpool: The Church of England Tent* and *The Church of England Tent, 39th Stationary Hospital, Ascq, September 1919*; William Orpen, *German Sick: Captured at Messines, in a Canadian Hospital.*

POETRY

Edmund Blunden, 'Vlamertinghe, Passing the Chateau, July 1917'.

10 Ambulance Trains

J. H. Plumridge's *Hospital Ships and Ambulance Trains*, (Seeley, Service & Co., 1975) is the main secondary source for details of this component of the military medical system. Plumridge describes the facilities on board the trains and how they were continually upgraded as the war went on. By 1917 the medical provision on ambulance trains, which included pharmacies, operating tables and sterilisation units, was comparable to that of CCSs. Treating ambulance trains as medical entities in their own right, rather than simply as links in a chain, would be a valuable approach in future research on the subject.

From the personal testimonies of ambulance-train staff we learn that the authority structure was minimal, with individual members taking a great deal of responsibility for the care of their patients. Unlike the nurses at the CCSs, those on ambulance trains were not able to develop specific technical skills beyond their general nursing training, but their work required considerable adaptation. Ambulance trains were often delayed and the wounded had to be kept calm and, if possible, happy. Staff and patients sat together for hours, and nurses devised ways of alleviating boredom and frustration. Staff came to identify closely with the train and their fellow crew members, and rich social lives developed. It does not appear that the train drivers and engineers were part of this social life, however, and further research would be needed to establish the reasons for this.

Leonard Horner's memoir is of particular value as it gives us insight into the world of the Friends' Ambulance Unit, a volunteer group formed by the pacifist Quakers. The Quaker movement's decision to offer their service of love in wartime is more complicated than it might seem. There were absolutists among them who refused to have anything to do with the war; they sought unconditional exemptions from mass conscription after 1916, and many of them went to prison. But the absolutists were in the minority: most Quakers worked from the very first days of the war to help its victims in Britain. Quaker organisations were among the first (and best organised) to offer aid to destitute refugees and enemy aliens. Later in the war they worked to help their fellow conscientious objectors, who often found themselves and their families in penury as a result of their principles. Other Quakers, such as Leonard Horner, were able to reconcile their pacifism with service at the front itself. Quakers joined non-combat units, such as the despatch riders, and medical services. In the process they saw the very worst of the war, up close and under fire.

Beyond his religious convictions, Horner may also be seen as representing a group of men and women who served in the war, but struggled to reconcile their principles with their work. Both at the front and back in Britain, medics questioned not only the war itself, but the role of medicine in furthering its aims and means. It was not just Quakers who had to make difficult decisions about their role in the war.

This chapter is based on the following primary sources: Miss Bickmore's 'Life on an Ambulance Train' (archives of the IWM, ref. 85/51/1); the personal archive of Nurse Morgan on No. 3 Train (IWM, ref. 06/100/1); the papers of Nurse Margaret Brander (IWM, ref. 05/06/1); and the papers of Leonard Horner (IWM, ref. GM62) The Quaker archives at Friends House in Euston Road, London are well organised and include both an excellent history of the FAU in *The Friends' Ambulance Unit: A Record* and a collection of No. 16's newsletters in *A Train Errant*. The archives contain many other personal memoirs of FAU members, which are yet to be explored.

REFERENCES

1   See the papers of Captain H. E. Meysey-Thompson, archives of the IWM, 92/19/1, entry for 21 September 1917.

2   See Catherine E. Hallett, *Containing Trauma: Nursing in the First World War* (Manchester University Press, 2009), p. 167.

3   See Captain H. C. Meysey-Thompson, archives of the IWM, 92/19/1.

4   See M. Tatham and J. E. Miles (eds), *The Friends' Ambulance Unit: A Record* (Strathmore Press, 1920), p. 149.

5   See John McCanley, 'A Manx Soldier's War Diary', for details of travel on the ambulance trains; McCanley papers in the archives of the IWM, 97/10/1. For McCanley, the journey had been tedious and painful.

6   See J. H. Plumridge, *Hospital Ships and Ambulance Trains.* (Seeley, Service & Co., 1975).

7   Tatham and Miles, *The Friends' Ambulance Unit*, p. 136.

8   See the collection of No. 16's newsletters in *A Train Errant*

(Simpson & Co, 1919). Newsletters and magazines written in hospitals and medical facilities were not limited to the front: see Jeffrey Reznick's *Healing the Nation: Soldiers and the Culture of Caregiving in Britain during the Great War* (Manchester University Press, 2004), pp. 65–98. There was greater censorship of magazines written and produced in hospitals in Britain, but the sense of humour was the same.

ART

John Lavery, *The Wounded at Dover*; Cecil Lawson, *Railway Station, Arras*; John Hodgson Lobley, *Loading Wounded at Boulogne*; Harold Septimus Power, *A Red Cross Train, France*.

POETRY

May Wedderburn Cannan, 'Rouen'; Wilfred Owen, 'The Send-Off'.

11 Furnes Railway Station

Studies of voluntarism and voluntary aid form a strong new historiographical strand in the history of the Great War. Works such as Jeffrey Reznick's *Healing the Nation* describe the range of voluntarist groups and their work with wounded soldiers, both in Britain and behind the front. Similarly, the work of the YMCA is described by Michael Snape in 'The Back Parts of War: The YMCA Memoirs and Letters of Barclay Baron, 1915 to 1919', *Church of England Record Society*, vol. 16, 2009. The YMCA also identified gaps in the evacuation system for the wounded in France. They put up a hut at Poperinghe Station, gave out hot drinks and food, and helped the men to write postcards home. They also installed teams at Le Havre, providing food, water and basic medical attention when the ambulance trains arriving from the Somme abandoned thousands of men on the platforms and docksides.

  Sarah MacNaughtan's work is part of this voluntarist tradition, but with one important distinction. She worked as an individual and was not part of any group, relying on no resources but her own. Such individuals could be found up and down the front, trying to find solutions for problems they had identified. They had certain features in common: they were usually rich enough to pay their own bills, of sufficient social and professional status to contemplate ignoring the authorities, and driven by an absolute commitment to their cause. Numerous such individuals contributed to the medical war. The dental surgeon Charles Valadier worked on Mickey Chater's facial injuries in a reconstructive unit that he had paid for himself. Elsie Knocker and Marie Chisholm, in their cellar house at Pervyse, ran their own aid post, without interference, until the building was destroyed by enemy shelling. Even so, MacNaughtan's story seems unique. The military authorities never interfered with her work at the railway station. She was able to take advantage of whatever part of the official military and medical infrastructure suited her: she was allowed to use the Red Cross delivery service to bring the supplies she had paid for across the Channel, even though she was not part of the Red Cross itself. She was not required to report to a male authority figure, in either the military or medical sphere. In short, she was given as much space as she needed and left to get on with it. It was only the failure of her own health that brought her work to an end.

The main source for Sarah MacNaughtan's work at Furnes Railway Station is her own memoir, *My War Experience on Two Continents*, which is available online or in printed form from Bibliobazaar. She also has an entry in the *Oxford Dictionary of National Biography*, by Harriet Blodgett, www.oxforddnb.com/view/article/59332/, accessed 17 August 2007. Her initiative and self-reliance were observed by others working at No. 1 Belgian Field, including Nurse Cora Mayne (archives of the IWM, no. 82/26/1).

ART

Christopher Nevinson, *La Patrie*.

12 Wounded

Joseph Pickard's testimony is drawn from his sound archive at the IWM (no. 8946). Details on the House of Hardy in the Great War are drawn from James Leighton Hardy's *The House the Hardy Brothers Built* (Medlar Press, 2006).

REFERENCES

1   A 'monkey jacket' was the equivalent of today's bomber jacket:
     a short jacket with elasticated cuffs and no collar, usually issued
     to Navy personnel. Pickard's would have come from a Red Cross
     store and was probably second-hand.

13 The London Ambulance Unit

The final chapter is drawn entirely from Claire Tisdall's 'Memoir of
the London Ambulance Column' (C. E. Tisdall, 1976; archives of the
IWM, no. 42 TIS). But for this memoir, the history of the LAC would
have faded away entirely, and this absence would have greatly diminished our understanding of the home front. All the Dent family papers
were destroyed in the Second World War and there is no mention of
them in the Red Cross archive. There is a brief reference in L/Cpl
Ward Muir's *Observations of an Orderly at an English War Hospital*
(Simpkin, Marshall, Hamilton & Kent, 1917) to 'that indefatigable body,
the London Ambulance Column'. Muir's memoirs are analysed in
Jeffrey Reznick's *Healing the Nation*, in the chapter 'Havens for Heroes'.

REFERENCES

1   There is some confusion as to the names of Mr and Mrs Dent.
     Miss Tisdall remembered the husband as Lancelot, but Mr Dent's
     school records have him as Lesley. As the archive of the Dent
     family business was destroyed, it has not been possible to be
     precise.
2   See The Nation's Fund for Nurses, archives of the Wellcome
     Trust, SA/NFN/C.1.2, p. 11.

ART

William Hatherell, *The Funeral Service of Edith Cavell at Westminster
Abbey, 15 May 1919*; Cecil Lawson, *Victory Parade*; John Hodgson Lobley,
*Outside Charing Cross Station, July 1916: Casualties from the Battle of the
Somme Arriving in London* and *Charing Cross Station: Detraining Wounded
by the British Red Cross Society and the Order of St John*.

POETRY

Wilfred Gibson, 'Bacchanal'; Robert Graves, 'Armistice Day'; Ivor Gurney, 'The Day of Victory'.

Epilogue

REFERENCES

1   See Michael Chater, *Family Business: A History of Grosvenor Chater, 1690–1977* (Grosvenor Chater & Co., 1977).

2   See the papers of Alfred Chater, archives of the IWM, 87/56/1, including 'A Harrow Memoir'.

3   See Charles Valadier, 'A Few Suggestions for the Treatment of Fractured Jaws', *British Journal of Surgery*, 1916, vol. IV, no. 13, pp. 64–73.

4   From conversations with the family of Bert Payne, in particular his granddaughter, the artist Sarah Pickstone, who won the 2013 John Moores Prize for painting.

5   Details of all post war medical careers were sourced from *The Medical Register*, copies covering the period from 1914 to 1965, consulted in the library of the Royal College of Surgeons.

6   Harold Gillies, *The Principles and Art of Plastic Surgery* (Butterworth, 1957), p. 23.

7   For details of William Kelsey Fry's work at Sidcup, see ibid. For Tonks's friendship with Kelsey Fry, see Joseph Hone, *The Life of Henry Tonks* (Heinemann, 1939), p. 130: 'In Kelsey Fry, the dental surgeon, one of Sir Harold's chief collaborators, Tonks also found a man of kindred tastes. To him he gave a gift of two small but accomplished works; in the first drawing, a piece of five figures, Sir Harold is seen operating, in the second (which is of considerable medical interest) a patient in the sitting position receives a general anaesthetic.'

8   The obituary of William Kelsey Fry in *The Lancet*, 2 November 1963, p. 954.

9   For the history of the Royal Victoria Hospital at Netley, see Philip Hoare, *Spike Island* (reissue; Fourth Estate, 2010).

10 Canon Ernest Crosse, sermon at Marlborough College, 25 May 1919, final page of transcript.

11   For details of all post-war ministries, see *Crockford's Clerical Directory*. Copy consulted in the Lambeth Palace Library, volumes for the period 1912 to 1970.

12   See *The War Letters of General Cyril Pereira to Henrietta Pereira, 1914–16*, vol. 1, entries for 4 March–1 October 1916. Both volumes are in the family's private collection, as is Father John's chalice.

13   Author's conversations with Father Timothy Radcliffe and Robin Baird-Smith, and private correspondence between Father John and Robin Baird-Smith, 12 April 1969.

Timeline

This timeline is for the Western Front of the Great War between 1914 and 1918. It is drawn primarily from John Keegan's *The First World War* (Pimlico, 1999) and Hew Strachan's *The First World War* (Simon & Schuster, 2003). For details of the Eastern Front, see Norman Stone's *The Eastern Front: 1914–1917* (Penguin, 1998), and for the Italian Front see Mark Thompson's *The White War: Life and Death on the Italian Front 1915–1919* (Faber and Faber, 2008)

In 1914, Europe divided into two coalitions. The Triple Entente comprised Russia, France and Great Britain. Germany was allied with the Habsburg Austro-Hungarian Empire. The main parties in the coalitions also had treaties with smaller European countries whose safety they guaranteed.

1914

28 June	Assassination in Serbia of Archduke Franz Ferdinand, nephew to the Emperor of Austria.
26–27 July	Serbia mobilises its army in response to Austrian diplomatic activity.
27 July	Russia mobilises in defence of Serbia.
28 July	Austria-Hungary declares war on Serbia.
1 August	Germany mobilises against Russia.
2 August	France mobilises against Germany.
4 August	Germany invades Belgium. Britain declares war on Germany in support of Belgium at midnight, after German failure to withdraw.
14 August	The Battle of the Frontiers begins: Britain, France and

	Germany engage each other along the French border.
21 August	Belgian army retreats to the entrenched camp at Antwerp.
23 August	Battle of Mons: British and French troops defeated.
24 August	French and British armies begin retreating along the entire length of the front. The end of the Battle of the Frontiers.
6 September	Retreat halted. Battle of the Marne begins. British and French troops hold the line and stop the German advance towards Paris.
9 September	German armies retreat back to a line along the River Aisne and begin to entrench. They hold most of Belgium and part of north-west France. This becomes known as the Flanders Position, where most of the fighting will take place over the next four years.
12 September	The 'Race for the Sea' begins as both sides turn north towards the Channel to secure a route to the coast. Entrenchment begins along the line.
22 September	No. 1 Belgian Field Hospital opens in Antwerp.
9 October	No. 1 Belgian Field Hospital evacuated from Antwerp.
10 October	Belgium surrenders, except for a small corner of territory behind a loop in the River Yser.
12 October	First battle of Ypres. Entrenched positions lengthen towards the coast. British and French forces plug the gap in the front, and German offensive fails.
21 October	No. 1 Belgian Field Hospital re-established at Furnes. **Henry Souttar** and **Sarah MacNaughtan** are on the staff.
10 November	**Jentie Patterson** writes her first letter to her sister, describing how No. 5 Casualty Clearing Station has become a front-line field hospital.
22 November	End of the battle of Ypres. High casualties on all sides and dreadful winter weather stop any significant offensive plans. Defensive positions ordered by both sides and trenches are dug in deep. The Western Front, as we now know it, is created.
29 November	Turkey attacks Russian Black Sea ports, joining the war on the side of Germany and Austria-Hungary.

8 December	**Sarah MacNaughtan** receives her specially made trolley from Harrods for her work at Furnes station.
14–24 December	First battle of Artois – inconclusive.
20 December	Smaller winter offensives are begun in Champagne by the French – inconclusive.

1915

Publication of the Oxford War Manuals begins.

3 January	Gas used by Germans at Bulimov on the Eastern Front.
10 March	Battle of Neuve Chapelle, first of the spring offensives.
12 March	**Mickey Chater** injured on last day of Neuve Chapelle. Battle ends inconclusively, but sets the pattern for future British and French offensives.
22 April	Germans use gas for the first time on the Western Front during the second battle of Ypres.
9 May	**William Kelsey Fry** wins Military Cross for bravery under fire retrieving casualties at Festubert.
23 May	Italy joins the war on the side of Britain, France and Russia.
25 May	End of second battle of Ypres.
May–June	Renewed offensives in Artois and Champagne.
1 June	**Sarah MacNaughtan** leaves Furnes and returns to England.
July	British troops reinforced.
25–28 September	Battle of Loos, part of the second offensive in Champagne. Frank Pierce, one of **William Kelsey Fry**'s bearers, wins the Distinguished Combat Medal. Father **John Lane Fox** buries men killed at the battle during the night. First British use of gas weapons.
13 October	Padre **Charles Doudney** killed by a shell.
6 November	End of British and French offensives on the Western Front.
6–8 December	Entente military commanders meet at Chantilly to

plan the great offensive for the forthcoming year, known as the Big Push.

1916

7 January	**William Kelsey Fry** refuses to leave his front-line RMO post for a casualty clearing station.
2 February	**Charles McKerrow** asks his wife to send him twenty pairs of medical scissors for his stretcher bearers.
21 February	German army begins new offensive at Verdun. It will grind on until December.
20 June	RMO **Geoffrey Hardwick** of 59th Field Ambulance charged extra for beer at the mess and told about the forthcoming Big Push by a local worker.
30 June	Padre **Ernest Crosse** builds medical posts with his RMO in preparation for the British and French offensive at the Somme.
1 July	Battle of the Somme begins. **Bert Payne**, the scout, injured at Montauban. The Royal Northumberland Fusiliers, with **Charles McKerrow** as RMO, are involved in the first day of the attack at La Boiselle: 2,440 men of the Northumberlands are killed, seventy from one small mining village alone.
7 July	RMO **Geoffrey Hardwick** notes 'Dead men + +' in his diary.
21 July	Padre **Ernest Crosse** leaves the Somme front line. Completes his grave map.
22 July	**Charles McKerrow** reports to his wife that three of his stretcher bearers have been given the Military Medal for their service during the Somme.
24 July	**Sarah MacNaughtan** dies in London.
29 August	**William Kelsey Fry** injured when his medical post is hit by a shell. Pearce and Sheasby from his bearer team are both killed.
19 November	End of the battle of the Somme. The two sides together have lost over a million men.

18 December	End of the battle of Verdun. German offensive pushed back.
20 December	RMO **Charles McKerrow** killed by a shell.

1917

6 April	America declares war on Germany.
9–15 April	Battle of Arras – inconclusive.
16 April–19 May	French offensives on the Aisne. All are inconclusive.
17 April	59th Field Ambulance hit by a shell. RMO **Geoffrey Hardwick** survives along with five bearers, but three others are killed. Padre **John Murray** takes up his front-line posting.
18 May	America enacts selective conscription for her armies.
7 June	British attack on Messines. German armies driven back and British armies gain a foothold.
4 July	First American units to arrive in France parade in Paris.
7 July	Air raid on No. 11 Casualty Clearing Station near Bailleul. Four doctors and twenty-three patients are killed; five doctors, sixty-three patients and the chaplain injured.
31 July	Third battle of Ypres begins (often called Passchendaele) to consolidate British gains.
21 August	**John Glubb** injured on the Hénin–Saint-Martin-sur-Cojeul road.
26 October	Russia, under her new communist leadership, leaves the war. German troops free to reinforce other fronts.
10 November	Dreadful weather and inconclusive results force the end of the battle of Passchendaele.
20–30 November	Battle of Cambrai. First significant use of tanks does not bring about a breakthrough.
23 December	Ambulance-train **Nurse Morgan** visits a battlefield and climbs a tank whilst her train spends Christmas in sidings in the middle of the trenches.

1918

21 March	First German offensive using reinforced Western Front army. Operation Michael attacks British army units on the old Somme battlefield.
1 April	Britain establishes the world's first independent air force, the RAF.
5 April	End of Michael offensive.
9 April	Germans launch Georgette offensive. Collapses after twelve-mile gain.
27 May	German Blücher offensive on the Aisne towards Paris begins.
6 June	Blücher offensive halted.
9 June	German Gneisenau offensive along River Matz.
14 June	Gneisenau offensive halted. American troops fight alongside French at Château-Thierry and Belleau Wood.
15 July	Last German offensive along Champagne–Marne line.
18 July	French and American troops halt the offensive in the second battle of the Marne.
19 July	German army begins retreat.
8 August	Battle of Amiens – significant victory for the Entente. German troops begin to surrender in large numbers.
30 August	First American Army fights near Verdun.
12 September	First all-American offensive of the war. German army falls back to 1914 positions.
26 September	Huge Entente offensive along the entire Western Front. German army retreats continually back into Germany.
30 October	Turkish Government asks for ceasefire.
3 November	Austrian Empire asks for ceasefire. Germany is the only power left fighting.
11 November	Armistice signed by Germany and Entente powers. The war is over.
12 November	Private Joseph Simpson dies in Nurse **Elizabeth Boon**'s ward.

Illustrations

Carrying wounded across the battlefield during the battle of Ginchy, 9 September 1916, © Imperial War Museums, Q1303.

Stretcher bearers carrying a wounded man over the top during the battle of Thiepval Ridge, September 1916, © Imperial War Museums, Q1332.

Bearers treating two soldiers at a dressing station during the battle of Pilckem Ridge, 31 July 1917, © Imperial War Museums, Q5732.

British doctor and padre attending to wounded British and Germans near Potijze, battle of the Menin Road, 20 September 1917, © Imperial War Museums, Q2857.

Wounded awaiting removal to a dressing station on the Menin Road, 20 September 1917. © Imperial War Museums, E711.

No. 44 Casualty Clearing Station at Puchevillers, photographed by the CCS's chaplain, Revd Leonard Pearson, © The Bodleian Library, University of Oxford.

Some of the staff at No. 44 Casualty Clearing Station, photographed by the CCS's chaplain, Revd Leonard Pearson, © The Bodleian Library, University of Oxford.

Field ambulance kit, © Science Museum / Science and Society Picture Library.

Field medical card of Sgt Thomas Riley, © the family of Thomas Riley, courtesy of Sylvia Riley.

Interior of a ward on a British ambulance train, near Doullens, 27 April 1918, © Imperial War Museums, Q8749.

Orderlies entraining a man wounded during the battle of Passchendaele, August 1917, © Imperial War Museums, CO1801.

Soldiers wounded during the battle of the Somme leaving Charing Cross Station, 8 July 1916, © Imperial War Museums, Q56277/Alfieri.

Bert Payne, © the Pickstone family, courtesy of Sarah Pickstone.

Charles Doudney, courtesy of Clive Castle and St Luke's Church, Bath.

Charles McKerrow in 1914, photography by William Crooke of Edinburgh © Imperial War Museums, Documents 2386.

Index

Printed in the USA/Agawam, MA
November 29, 2023

855911.067